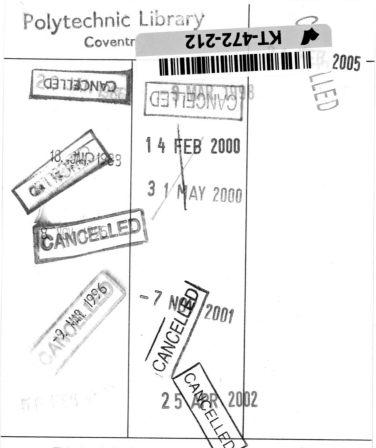

Disease in African History

The Committee on Commonwealth and Comparative Studies of Duke University

Ralph Braibanti

John W. Cell

R. Taylor Cole

Craufurd D. W. Goodwin

Gerald W. Hartwig

Richard H. Leach, *Vice Chairman*

Richard A. Preston

A. Kenneth Pye, *Chairman*

Frank T. de Vyver, *Secretary-Treasurer*

Disease in African History

An Introductory Survey and Case Studies

Mario Joaquim Azevedo   James W. Brown
Mark W. DeLancey   Charles M. Good
Gerald W. Hartwig   K. David Patterson

Edited by
Gerald W. Hartwig
and
K. David Patterson

Number 44 in a series published for the
Duke University Center for Commonwealth and Comparative Studies
Duke University Press, Durham, N.C.
1978

© 1978 Duke University Press

L.C.C. card no. 78–52421

I.S.B.N. 0–8223–0410–4

Printed in the United States of
America by Kingsport Press, Inc.

To our parents

Faith L. and Walter A. Hartwig

and

Elizabeth C. and Karl D. Patterson

Preface

In the fall of 1974 the editors of this volume discovered that they shared an interest in the role of disease and medicine in African history. One of us (Gerald W. Hartwig) presented a paper on disease and long-distance trade at the annual meeting of the African Studies Association; the other (K. David Patterson) published a bibliographical essay surveying the existing literature on the subject. Informal soundings showed that a number of Africanists, particularly in the Southeast, shared the same interest. Under the leadership of Gerald Hartwig, a Symposium on Disease and History in Africa was subsequently held at the Quail Roost Conference Center in April 1975. All of the contributors to this volume participated; several presented early versions of the essays appearing here.

This volume does not pretend to give a complete or systematic survey of the vast and almost uncharted field of disease in the history of Africa. Such a synthesis will not be possible until much more research is done. The individual essays, reflecting the diverse interests and approaches of their authors as well as the limitations of the various types of sources, have raised a multitude of questions but few reassuring answers; the following case-studies clearly illustrate problems and possibilities for further research. Our main purpose, addressed in the introduction, is to demonstrate the vital importance of health and disease in understanding Africa's past.

We are grateful to Dr. John W. Cell of Duke University and Dr. Gert Brieger, formerly of Duke University and now of the Department of History of Health Sciences at the University of California, San Francisco, who served as commentators at the Quail Roost session. Dr. Brieger's advice and enthusiasm as a medical historian were especially welcome as we entered what we saw as a highly technical and intimidating field. We are particularly indebted to John Cell for his continuing encouragement of the project as well as his sharp editorial eye. We would also like to express our appreciation to Dr. Robert Mundt of the University of North Carolina at Charlotte for reading and commenting on various essays, to Kathleen A. Sharp for her excellent editing work, and to Eloise H. Webster for the patience and endurance required in preparing the manuscript for press. Of course, none of these colleagues and friends are responsible for remaining shortcomings.

Contributors

Mario Joaquim Azevedo, Associate Professor of History, Jackson State University. He received his doctorate from Duke University in 1975. His research has been on the Sara of southern Chad. His major concern has been on demographic conditions, including the effects of labor migration as well as epidemic disease, during the present century.

James W. Brown, Associate Professor of History, University of South Carolina at Spartanburg. His primary research interest has been on social and economic history in an urban setting, specifically on Kumasi in south central Ghana. The study necessarily included aspects of health and disease during the twentieth century. In 1972 he received his Ph.D. from the University of Wisconsin, Madison.

Mark W. DeLancey, Associate Professor, Department of Government and International Studies, University of South Carolina at Columbia. In 1973 he received his Ph.D. in Political Science from Indiana University. His interest in health conditions emanated from his research on migration and ethnicity in Cameroon. Recently he has been conducting research on Nigerian domestic and international politics.

Charles M. Good, Professor of Geography and Chairman of the Department, Virginia Polytechnic Institute and State University. In 1970 he received his doctorate from University of Chicago. He has conducted research in Uganda and, more recently, Kenya. He is basically a medical geographer whose interests range from the historical interrelationship between economic activities and disease to the spatial aspects of health care delivery.

Gerald W. Hartwig, Professor of History, Duke University. He received his Ph.D. from Indiana University in 1971. In addition to medical history, which emerged as a crucial element in the understanding of the nineteenth century in East Africa, his research interests include economic and social changes since 1800. He has conducted extensive research in Tanzania and is currently examining health-related topics in Sudan.

K. David Patterson, Associate Professor of History, University of North Carolina at Charlotte. He received his Ph.D. from Stanford University in 1971. His initial research was focused on economic activities along the coast of northern Gabon where he learned the significance of health factors in historical studies. His work now revolves around disease and health care in Ghana where he has conducted research during the past three years.

Contents

Tables, Maps, and Figures

Disease in African History

The Disease Factor: An Introductory Overview

K. David Patterson and Gerald W. Hartwig

Historians of Africa have generally neglected the study of past health conditions—as well as the role of disease, health care, and medicine in history—despite the obvious importance of the disease burden on the African continent. Major epidemics, which have often accompanied ecological change, migration, or foreign contacts, have tested institutions and decimated populations. A host of endemic afflictions have restricted settlement of large areas, sapped the strength and shortened the lives of Africans, and limited their productivity. For centuries, the continent's disease environment contributed to its relative isolation from non-African civilizations.

The intrinsic importance of the subject cannot be denied, but the historical study of health and disease forces the scholar to consider a society in its total cultural and environmental setting, a detailed and demanding task. For this reason it is encouraging that Africanists as well as historians and specialists in other areas are now showing signs of interest in the significance of disease's historical role.[1] Our intention in this book is to illustrate the importance of health-related issues in African history, to encourage scholars to examine or at least to be aware of the disease factor within their own chronological and geographical specialties, and to suggest specific problems and topics requiring significantly more research.

Most human societies normally exist in some sort of rough equilibrium with their pathogens—the specific causes of their diseases—adapting to their disease environment in a number of biological and cultural ways. They may develop genetic defenses over generations, such as sickle cell trait which provides some protection against malaria. And, since a parasite which is too virulent endangers its own survival by destroying its potential hosts, selective pressures tend to produce more moderate pathogens. Exposure to most diseases stimulates the body's immunological defenses, which provides protection of varying degree and duration.[2] Cultural responses are equally important. Societies typically have some functionally useful standards of personal and community cleanliness. Medical techniques are developed in an attempt to control the incidence and severity of various diseases. People learn to avoid certain sources of danger, such as tsetse-infested bush, polluted water, or unnecessary contact with victims of diseases they think are contagious.

These protective mechanisms have been only partially effective. African disease environments, frequently augmented by tropical climatic conditions, have always exacted a significant toll on human life and energy. But, unless man/parasite-vector relationships were altered by such factors as contacts with strangers and their diseases, changes in settlement patterns, movement into a new ecological zone, alteration in modes of transportation, or dramatic change in life-styles, the epidemiological and demographic situation could be expected to remain roughly stable. Epidemic outbreaks would be unusual, but endemic afflictions were common enough and, while frequently chronic in adults, caused high mortality among infants and toddlers. A long-standing cultural premium on fertility and childbearing produced birth rates sufficiently high to balance or slightly exceed Africa's seemingly high death rates before 1945.[3] The assumption that death rates in the precolonial era, or more precisely, the era before extensive contact with aliens, were as high as those of the earlier colonial period is probably incorrect. With the apparent partial exception of West Africa, the unhealthiest period in all African history was undoubtedly between 1890 and 1930.

Conditions of relative equilibrium between man and his diseases have been broken and restored several times in the course of African history. Village agriculture, trade contacts with Europeans and Asians, and the establishment of colonial rule all created new and more complex disease environments for African peoples. These changes took place at different times in various parts of the continent, with West Africans generally experiencing them earlier than inhabitants of other areas, with the exception of North Africa. Because of this fact and because accommodation to new conditions took place at differing rates, it is likely that epidemiological conditions varied widely from region to region at any given time.

Early hunting and gathering peoples had millenia to achieve biological harmony with their microbial and helminthic parasites. The advent of settled village life broke this balance. Economies based on agriculture or intensive fishing could support larger groups of people in relatively fixed places. Concentrated populations created, for the first time in man's evolution, favorable conditions for the spread of acute viral diseases such as smallpox, measles, poliomyelitis, influenza, and the many varieties of the common cold. Infection conveys long-lasting immunity against that specific viral strain to the survivors, and, since these viruses do not persist in a latent state in their hosts and have no animal reservoir, they can survive only by continual transfer from victims to nonimmune persons. Therefore, these diseases required more hosts than a hunting and gathering economy could support and must have first afflicted man after what we refer to as the Neolithic Revolution.[4] Village life also caused the appearance or at least a dramatic increase in enteric diseases such as amoebic and bacillary dysentery and typhoid fever. Such diseases of the alimentary system are acquired by drinking water contaminated with human wastes. Large numbers of people living in close contact thus provided a critical mass of potential hosts and enhanced the opportunities for infection with organisms transmitted by the respiratory and the fecal-oral routes.[5] Conditions for the transmission of water-borne helminthic diseases such as guinea worm and schistosomiasis were also enhanced. In addition, new methods of food production increased exposure to a variety of pathogens. Domestic animals harbored flukes, roundworms, tapeworms, and micro-organisms dangerous to man, in addition to ticks which served as vectors for relapsing fever and some rickettsial diseases.[6] Clearing forests for agriculture created favorable breeding conditions for *Anopheles gambiae,* the mosquito which is the primary vector of falciparum malaria.[7] Wet rice cultivation and irrigation exposed farmers to schistosomiasis, a fluke which requires certain freshwater snails as an intermediate host.

The price Africans paid for the benefits of more efficient food production and settled village life was a more complex and threatening disease environment. Quite possibly, some of these by-products of a new civilization accompanied or preceded the movements of Bantu-speaking people into central, eastern, and southern Africa. If so, alien diseases weakened the ability of the aboriginal pygmoid and Khoisan-speaking inhabitants to resist Bantu expansion.[8] As was the case in the Western Hemisphere after 1492, disease may have been an ally of conquerors.

Most African societies experienced many centuries of relative isolation between the rise of village agriculture and their first contact with non-Africans and their diseases. During this period, which lasted well into the nineteenth century in some regions, people developed natural and cultural defenses against local strains of pathogens. Technological conservatism and manageable rates of population growth—emigration being a frequent means of adapting to an increase in numbers—minimized the likelihood of sudden ecological changes which might disturb the relationships between humans, parasites, and vectors. The extent of interaction with neighboring communities varied greatly from place to place and over time, but almost everywhere commercial and other contacts were much less frequent or intense than they have become during the last century or so. Even where long-distance trade had a substantial history, as in parts of West Africa, the impact on the disease environment might well have been more limited than normally expected. Small groups of merchants followed well-defined routes on a seasonal basis and probably had little contact with people living even a few miles off the roads. Further, some long-distance trade involved relatively little human movement because specific communities prohibited transit traffic. Instead, these communities acquired goods on one frontier and carried what they did not want to keep across their own territory to exchange with yet another neighboring community. Such practices reduced the possibility that contagious diseases would spread over large areas. It seems reasonable to postulate that traditional "precontact" Africa suffered relatively few major epidemics. Natural barriers such as oceans and deserts, combined with slow communication, prevented most epidemics from reaching sub-Saharan Africa. Endemic diseases and natural disasters such as droughts and locust invasions, however, certainly affected population growth.

Many African disease environments were extremely dangerous for outsiders. Europeans, whether traders, explorers, soldiers, missionaries, or would-be "civilizers" like the participants in the Niger expedition of 1841, generally found Africa's "fevers" and "fluxes" deadly until the beginning of tropical medicine in the late nineteenth century.[9] With the significant exception of specific climatic regions found in extreme North and South Africa, early European activity was limited by exceedingly high death rates.[10] The claim of a French trader that parts of the Guinea Coast were so unhealthy that the slave trade there was "an exchange of whites for blacks"[11] was a gross exaggeration, but the point made is understandable. The continent's epidemiological barriers also proved formidable for settlers of African descent who had lost their ancestors' immunity to tropical diseases while in North America and who found the disease environment very hazardous in Sierra Leone and Liberia.[12] North African merchants suffered from local diseases in the Western Sudan,[13] and visitors to the Swahili Coast no doubt had comparable problems. Africa's epidemiological environment has played a major role in the relative isolation of the continent throughout most of its history.

Despite these hazards, foreigners came to Africa and, by bringing their own diseases with them, disrupted the existing equilibrium. Intensifying commercial and military contacts between Africans and foreigners—be they Europeans, North Africans, Arabs, or Africans from distant places—breached previously isolated disease environments. In Africa, as in the Americas, the Pacific Islands, and elsewhere, the breakdown of isolation meant the introduction of new pathogens and new strains of familiar bacteria, protozoa, and viruses. Major epidemics resulted, with substantial population losses.[14]

Although as we have said many regions remained relatively isolated until the nineteenth century, the introduction of cosmopolitan diseases into Africa took place over a thousand year period. Trading communities in the grasslands of western Africa and the East African coast had almost certainly been affected by 1000 A.D. Africans along the western coast encountered disease-bearing Europeans during the second half of the fifteenth century; the inhabitants of the Zambezi valley met them after 1500, and Khoisan peoples[15] in southern Africa after the mid-seventeenth century. We know very little about the epidemiological and demographic consequences of these early contacts, but Muslim and European travelers must have introduced Africans they encountered to diseases such as smallpox, measles, and syphilis by 1600. From what is known from other world communities, it is logical to assume that there was significant depopulation in specific areas as a result of these early contacts, even if the extreme aboriginal death rates of the Caribbean were not replicated.

In western Africa, maritime and trans-Saharan commerce encouraged a steady growth of long-distance trade. Increased intercommunication, combined with political upheavals in some areas, as among the Akan states, facilitated the spread of introduced diseases into the interior. It is reasonable to assume that most communities in this region suffered the initial consequences of epidemiological change at a relatively early date. During the nineteenth and early twentieth centuries, West Africans did not experience the same catastrophic epidemics and depopulation common elsewhere in the continent, despite an expansion of trade and political unrest in many places.[16] By 1800 West Africans had had many generations to build up defenses to cope with their more complex disease environment, though such defenses were, of course, only partial. For example, ships periodically brought in smallpox, and whenever enough time had passed between introductions for a new generation of previously unexposed and therefore nonimmune people to appear, major epidemics with high mortality reoccurred. Despite the apparent antiquity of indigenous forms of variolization, smallpox remained a serious menace well into the twentieth century.[17]

The movement of diseases was not a one-way process. Europe and the Americas acquired deadly yellow fever epidemics from West Africa, and the slave trade was responsible for the transmission of many helminthic infections, including hookworm, filariasis, and onchocerciasis, into the New World. African strains of malaria and dysentery played a major role in early American demographic history, especially among the Indians in the lowlands of the Caribbean basin.[18] Even in the temperate climate of Britain's North American colonies, African diseases killed thousands of the white population, partially offsetting the overall population growth resulting from the importation of Africans.[19]

Interaction with alien disease environments took place much later in most of the interior of eastern and equatorial Africa. Here, in contrast to West Africa, recurrent and often devastating epidemics characterized the nineteenth and early twentieth centuries and, in many areas, caused substantial depopulation.[20] The expansion of trade and the rise of secondary empires provided ideal conditions for the spread of disease.[21] Caravans, frequently consisting of hundreds of participants, traveled hundreds of miles inland. Elephant hunters and slave-raiders operated over large areas, destroying or confiscating crops, disrupting societies, and forcing thousands to flee into tsetse-infested bush or malarial lowlands. Famine was not an uncommon threat.[22] Even victorious groups could wind up in unhealthy places. The Kololo, a Sotho group displaced during the Mfecane, gained control over Lozi country in the Zambezi floodplain in the 1830s. By 1865, however, they had lost their dominant political position partly because malaria, an unfamiliar disease, had badly weakened them.

Psychological stress can reduce resistance to infection, and for many East Africans the collapse of familiar institutions and the dangerously fluid social and political situation must have produced tremendous stress.[23] Uprooted, malnourished populations proved terribly vulnerable to major killers like smallpox, cholera, and later trypanosomiasis. Measles and other diseases, including the great rinderpest epizootic which decimated herds in the 1880s and 1890s,[24] contributed to the general misery. The jigger or sand flea, *Tunga penetrans*, an annoying and potentially dangerous pest, was introduced from Brazil to Angola about 1850. Thanks to increased intercommunication, the insect had spread over most of tropical Africa by the early 1890s.

The contrasts between nineteenth-century West Africa, where some biological defenses had developed by 1800, and most of the rest of the continent are striking, but the consequences of the spread of Eurasian diseases were probably equally devastating. Calamitous "virgin soil" epidemics and the most epidemiologically destructive consequences of state formation and slaving took place earlier in West Africa and were largely beyond the ken of literate observers. European records and indigenous Islamic writings will provide some clues if the proper questions are asked,[25] but our knowledge of the demographic and social consequences of epidemiological change will certainly be less adequate for West Africa than for areas which suffered later.

Africans dealt with the crisis of a suddenly much more complex disease environment in various ways. Certainly, they were much more successful than most American Indian, Polynesian, Melanesian, or Australian Aboriginal groups. The reasons for this are not clear, but, perhaps because of lesser isolation and hence an ancient partial overlap in disease environments, Africans had greater resistance to Eurasian diseases. Perhaps African societies responded better to the stress of widespread illness, providing better care of the sick and avoiding economic collapse. Also, the fact that many African societies had less direct European pressure at the time of epidemiological crisis may have been significant. In any case, even when decimated and displaced, most African groups showed considerable resilience. Selective pressures encouraged the development of degrees of immunity to various diseases. Indigenous therapeutic practices, including herbal medicines and variolization, were sometimes useful. Families, lineages, and ethnic groups sometimes tried to make up for population loss by incorporating outsiders in a servile capacity, or as clients, or as wives.[26] This phenomenon seems to have been widespread during the nineteenth century and probably earlier whenever conditions encouraged it. The necessity of replacing victims of epidemic diseases probably played a contributory role in the evolution of many African systems of servitude. Witchcraft, sorcery, and witchcraft eradication movements must also be examined to determine their potential and probable relationship to an altering disease environment.[27]

The disorders caused by the colonial conquest of the late nineteenth century, a continuation of previous turmoil in some places, provided further opportunities for the spread of diseases. European troops introduced diseases, and they themselves contracted considerable sickness, despite the major advances of quinine and boiled drinking water. In any case, colonial armies employed large numbers of African soldiers, and military units, supported by long columns of porters, crisscrossed the countryside, carrying with them respiratory and intestinal diseases associated with camp life. The use of river routes helped spread virulent strains of trypanosomes, especially in equatorial Africa. Both colonial and African forces lived off the land and in some areas of heavy fighting, as in French campaigns against Samori Toure, famine and disease went hand in hand.

Colonial rule had a profound impact on the health of Africans and, indeed, has largely created the continent's present disease environment. Government policies and African responses to them often inadvertently created conditions favorable to the spread of disease. On the other hand, European colonial regimes also introduced modern preventive and curative medicine to the continent.

All colonial governments tried to improve transportation networks. Efficient movement of people and goods was essential for administrative control and economic exploitation of the newly acquired territories. Internal trade barriers were eliminated and banditry suppressed. Roads, railways, and harbors were built and greater use was made of navigable waterways. The advent of motor vehicles shortly before World War I was a major stimulus for trade and mobility. Steamships carried plague and influenza from port to port. Clearly, greater intercommunication meant a more rapid spread of disease. On a continental scale, the rapid

spread of influenza in 1918–19 was made possible by the developing transportation network.[28] Cerebrospinal meningitis periodically swept the Sahel region south of the Sahara.[29] Short-distance
mobility was often sufficient to introduce people to new strains
of familiar diseases, as Good's chapter in this volume shows for
tick-borne relapsing fever. Intensified interaction within regions
must have disturbed the relative tolerance which many rural
Africans had acquired for local strains of the parasites causing
malaria, dysentery, trypanosomiasis, and perhaps other indigenous diseases.[30]

The epidemiological importance of greater intercommunication
is obvious, but it is difficult to deal with on other than a very
general level. Clearly, there was more intercommunication in,
say, 1930 than in 1830, but how much more and how can it be
measured? Distance of movements, the ecological zones crossed,
the number of people moving, the nature of their contacts with
population en route and at their destination, and the previous
disease exposure of the groups involved are among the variables
which must be considered. Intercommunication had different
effects on different occupational and ethnic groups. Traders who
traveled long distances and their commercial contacts and hosts
encountered a greater risk of disease than subsistence farmers
dwelling some distance away from roads or major trade centers.
In West Africa, where women do much of the local marketing,
females would presumably have experienced increased risk. Exposure to disease would vary among ethnic as well as occupational groups in accordance with their mobility and participation
in commerce.

Colonial economic policies often had serious consequences for
human health, as Azevedo's investigation of the Sara indicates.
Forced labor existed at various times in all colonies, and had the
potential to disrupt agriculture and to move people into unfamiliar disease environments. Mark DeLancey's essay on German labor policies in Cameroon is an excellent case in point.
Other flagrant and devastating examples include the French por-
terage system between the basins of the Ubangui and Chari

rivers and forced rubber collection in equatorial forest zones controlled by France and by Leopold of Belgium.

Taxation of Africans was frequently designed to channel labor from subsistence agriculture to enterprises of interest to colonial governments. Construction, cash crop production, and mining required large numbers of unskilled workers who could be readily produced by levying head or hut taxes payable in cash. Labor migration, whether a voluntary reaction to economic opportunity or a necessary response to rural poverty and taxation, had major implications for health. The migrants, generally poor, ragged, and badly nourished, often walked or rode hundreds of miles, bringing their own diseases with them. At their destination, they encountered hostile local disease environments and faced additional hazards inherent in their marginality and in their new occupations. Migrants to urban areas frequently had to live in crowded squalor where they were vulnerable to a variety of respiratory and enteric diseases. Lumber workers were frequently exposed to harsh conditions to remote forest camps. Returning migrants brought their newly acquired afflictions back to their rural homelands. Syphilis in northern Ghana was called the 'Kumasi Sickness' for good reason; tuberculosis was spread in that country and in southern Africa by discharged miners.[31]

Agricultural policies, especially the encouragement of cash crop production for export, influenced health conditions in a number of ways. Plantations and small African producers required seasonal migrant labor. Also colonial agriculture had an impact on nutrition, a subject requiring extensive examination. Resources devoted to commercial crops had to be diverted from food crops, and the nutritional consequences of decreased food production may or may not have been balanced by greater ability to purchase food. Monoculture of cotton or peanuts led to widespread soil exhaustion, while agricultural research was largely confined to crops raised for sale on the world market. On the other hand, colonial animal husbandry and veterinary efforts helped increase the quality and quantity of cattle, sheep, goats, swine, and poultry, thus making animal protein more readily available. Clearing forests for cocoa farms created favorable breeding conditions for *A. gambiae,* a major malaria vector. Dams and irrigation projects designed to increase agricultural productivity were often more successful in spreading diseases. Dam ponds increased exposure to mosquito-borne diseases and to guinea worm; irrigation ditches provided habitats for the snail vectors of schistosomiasis, a disease which has spread rapidly in twentieth-century Africa.[32]

The dangers of well-intentioned but ill-informed rural development schemes is illustrated by the following tale, which describes events in Kenya between 1957 and 1961.

Once upon a time (but not too long ago) there lived a tribe deep within the Dark Continent. These people tilled the soil to raise crops of roots and grains, for they had little meat to lend them strength. Illness often befell them, but even so, in this dry land they were not overly troubled with the fever sickness brought by the mosquito. Now in the Northern World there was a powerful republic that had compassion on these people and sent their Wise Men to relieve the mean burden of their lives. The Wise Men said, "Let them farm fish," and taught the people to make ponds and to husband a fish called tilapia.

The people learned well, and within a short time they had dug 10,000 pits and ponds. The fish flourished, but soon the people could not provide the constant labors required to feed the fish and keep the ponds free of weeds. The fish became smaller and fewer, and into these ponds and pits came the fever mosquitoes, which bred and multiplied prodigiously. The people then sickened and the children died from the fever that the medicine men from the cities called malaria. The Wise Men from the North departed, thinking how unfortunate it was that these people could not profit from their teachings. The people of the village thought it strange that Wise Men should be sent them to instruct in the ways of growing mosquitoes.[33]

Colonial governments, by accident or design, often had a major impact on settlement patterns. People increasingly chose, or were required, to live in larger villages or along roads, rather than in scattered hamlets. These conditions obviously facilitated the transmission of disease. On the other hand, population pressures and official policies often encouraged the colonization of new lands. In the bush, especially along rivers, people were frequently placed in closer contact with the vectors of *Trypanosoma gambiense* and *T. rhodesiense,* the protozoa which cause sleeping sickness.

Urbanization, a recent phenomenon in much, although certainly not all of the continent, was a vital factor in the creation of modern disease environments. Cities, magnets for migrants and the hubs of the transportation systems, were foci for the diffusion of disease. And, in Africa as elsewhere, crowded urban conditions proved ideal breeding grounds for respiratory and enteric diseases. Sewerage, water supplies, refuse collection, and housing lagged far behind the needs of the rising tide of migrants. Still, enough modern sanitary and medical technology was introduced to alleviate many of the health problems associated with rapid urbanization. In contrast to the demographic costs of early urbanization in Europe, twentieth-century African cities have had significantly lower death rates than the countryside. The medical and demographic implications of preindustrial urbanization are of general significance in world history and, as African cities have developed relatively recently and data is more abundant than, for example, seventeenth-century Europe, studies of these urban problems in Africa should be of wide interest.[34]

Thus, the colonial period and its accompanying changes unleashed serious health problems in Africa. Plague, tuberculosis, pneumonia, dysentery, and other diseases affected urban areas; smallpox, measles, syphilis, gonorrhea, tick and louse-borne relapsing fevers, cerebrospinal meningitis, influenza, and the other infections spread more easily, and familiar diseases like malaria, schistosomiasis, and trypanosomiasis could claim more victims.

By introducing modern medical technology and by encouraging research in the developing field of tropical medicine, however, colonialism contributed to the control of the epidemiological problems it helped to create. Public health and medical measures began to counteract the outburst of communicable diseases which characterized the first decades of the colonial era. By c. 1920–30 the demographic decline experienced by many people was halted and accelerating population growth became the norm. The relative contributions of medical measures and rising standards of living to mortality reduction are still unclear, but in Africa it

seems probable that preventive and curative medicine played a
larger role than in industrial countries.[35] Rapid population growth
may prove to be one of the major legacies of the latter part of the
colonial period.

Colonial medical services have been the subject of much more
discussion than serious research. Early medical staffs were clearly
inadequate in numbers and in quality, even by the meager standards of Africa today. Funding was chronically inadequate. Even
in the French colonies, where serious efforts were made to serve
rural areas, medical facilities were concentrated in large towns.
Medical departments were often surprisingly unaware of the extent or even the existence of some major problems, as Patterson's
chapter on onchocerciasis in the Gold Coast and Hartwig's discussion of relapsing fever in Sudan demonstrate. Even when diseases
were recognized and their ecology understood, preventive measures were often almost impossible. Smallpox vaccination campaigns were hindered by rapid deterioration of vaccine in tropical
conditions. Quarantines frequently failed to control outbreaks.
Malaria, dysentery, guinea worm, hookworm, and many other
chronic conditions could not be controlled without major socioeconomic changes in the countryside. Therapeutic measures were
often ineffective or unknown until late in the colonial period.
Arsenic and bismuth compounds were used with some success
against syphilis, yaws, relapsing fever, and sleeping sickness in
the 1920s, but serious side effects sometimes plagued mass treatment campaigns. Otherwise, except for quinine, used as a specific
drug against malaria from the 1840s, and emetine for amoebic
dysentery, drugs effective against microorganisms were almost
nonexistent. Indeed, not until the development of sulpha drugs
in the mid-1930s and antibiotics during World War II could physicians directly attack most pathogenic bacteria. Cheap, effective
drug therapy, the only hope for the rapid alleviation of mass
illness in poor tropical countries, was only possible in the last 15
or 20 years of colonial rule.[36]

The achievements of colonial medical departments were limited by their priorities and goals, as well as by limits on staffs,
funding, and knowledge. The protection of European health was

factors. An examination of the role of health care, disease, medicine, and nutrition will enhance the value of their own work and will provide data for scholars directly concerned with medical questions.

Studies are needed on many specific problems. The role of disease as an isolating factor in African history deserves a great deal more attention, particularly as it influenced interactions of people on either side of the Sahara Desert and the interactions of indigenous people and traders along the East African coast. The precolonial impact of Eurasian diseases remains largely unknown. Studies on specific epidemics and diseases are essential. An epidemic is a time of testing for a society's political, economic, social, and cultural institutions, so societal responses to epidemics must be examined as well as the demographic consequences;[40] Hartwig's contribution on social consequences of disease in East Africa confronts these developments and suggests one way to understand societal responses. Influenza probably killed at least two million Africans during the 1918–19 pandemic, but our knowledge of this catastrophe and its effect upon the survivors is still meager. The sleeping sickness epidemic in Uganda in the early twentieth century has been examined but, despite some suggestive work, we know little about its apparently equally devastating impact in former French Equatorial Africa.[41] Tuberculosis and venereal diseases also deserve historical study, and research is needed on the difficult topic of nutritional changes in response to new food crops, commercial agriculture, imported canned foods, and the production and trading of fish and livestock. Urban health, both precolonial and modern, is a fertile field for future scholarship, as is the impact of improved transportation systems upon disease environments. The competence, capabilities, strategies, and effectiveness of colonial medical services must be examined in the context of the political-social situation and the development of scientific tropical medicine. Dentistry, the incidence and treatment of mental illness, medical education, nursing, rural health care, and the use of paramedical personnel should be studied. Research on colonial health care systems could shed valuable light on current problems. Intercolonial cooperation on health matters, or the lack of it,[42] deserves attention, as do the activities of the international agencies such as the World Health Organization and the League of Nations Epidemiological Service. Veterinary medicine, apparently one of the most successful activities of colonial governments, has received almost no attention. Little historical writing has been done on changes in African attitudes toward disease, the evolution of indigenous healing systems, African responses to modern medicine and its practitioners, or the political implications of health-related issues. Finally, demographic history is now beginning to interest Africanists.[43] The impact of epidemic disease and modern medicine on population changes in the last century or so is a compelling topic for future investigation.

The field of African history has developed extraordinarily rapidly during the past two decades. As the scope and sophistication of research increase, medical and disease factors should become more prominent. Historians of Africa, generally not the sort of people who fear interdisciplinary approaches, need not be intimidated by the technical nature of the subject. None of the contributors to this volume has had specialized medical training. The medical literature is accessible through an impressive array of bibliographical tools.[44] Data on medical topics are often sparse, scattered, and of doubtful quality, but this is hardly a novel problem for Africanists. A willingness to read, consult standard reference works, and ask questions, as well as a realistic sense of one's limits are of course necessary, as would be true for studies using tools and concepts from archeology, linguistics, social anthropology, or any other discipline.

A holistic approach is essential for the study of the historical role of disease and medicine. Since health conditions are a function of the total natural and social environment, the historian must deal with the entire ecological situation of a people. Agriculture, economics, housing, settlement patterns, demographic composition, social organization, cultural and religious values, medical technology, political conditions, epidemiological history, nutrition, climate, vegetation, fauna, topography, and other factors all influence the host-parasite relationship, and often, vice versa. Research on changing health conditions may lead the investigator inexorably into fields as diverse as forestry, religion, geography, social anthropology, veterinary medicine, or demography. For scholars concerned with human health, history can never be reduced to past politics.

Notes

1. Philip Curtin, Steven Feierman, Leonard Thompson, and Jan Vansina, *African History* (Boston, 1978), pp. 552–55; K. David Patterson, "Disease and Medicine in African History: A Bibliographical Essay," *History in Africa*, I (1974), 141–48. Useful works by physicians on the relationships between health conditions and history include Hans Zinsser, *Rats, Lice, and History* (New York, 1935, and many subsequent editions); Henry E. Sigerist, *Civilization and Disease* (Ithaca, N.Y., 1943; Chicago, 1970); Frederick F. Cartwright, *Disease and History* (New York, 1974); and Thomas McKeown, *The Modern Rise of Population* (New York, 1976). Suggestive recent works by historians include two books by Alfred W. Crosby, *The Columbian Exchange: The Biological Consequences of 1492* (Westport, Conn., 1972) and *Epidemic and Peace, 1918* (Westport, Conn., 1976), and William H. McNeill, *Plagues and Peoples* (New York, 1976).

2. Lucid introductions to disease ecology are available in Sir Macfarlane Burnet and David O. White, *Natural History of Infectious Disease* (Cambridge, U.K., 1972) and Rene Dubos, *Man Adapting* (New Haven, 1965).

3. John C. Caldwell, "Introduction," in J. C. Caldwell, ed., *Population Growth and Socioeconomic Change in West Africa* (New York, 1975), p. 4.

4. Francis L. Black, "Infectious Diseases in Primitive Societies," *Science*, CLXXXVII (14 February 1975), 515–18.

5. Frank Fenner, "The Effects of Changing Social Organisation on the Infectious Diseases of Man," in S. V. Boyden, ed., *The Impact of Civilisation on the Biology of Man* (Toronto, 1970), pp. 49–68.

6. Geoffrey Lapage, *Animals Parasitic in Man* (New York, 1963) is a useful introduction to medical parasitology.

7. For the relationships between agriculture, malaria, and sickle-cell trait, see Stephen L. Wiesenfeld, "Sickle-Cell Trait in Human Biological and Cultural Evolution," *Science*, CLVII (8 September 1967), 1134–40.

8. This idea was suggested to us by Philip Curtin at the African Studies Association Meeting in Boston, November 1976.

9. Philip D. Curtin, *The Image of Africa: British Ideas and Action, 1780–1850* (Madison, 1964), pp. 177–97, 343–62.

10. K. G. Davies, "The Living and the Dead: White Mortality in West Africa, 1684–1732," in Stanley L. Engerman and Eugene D. Genovese, eds., *Race and Slavery in the Western Hemisphere: Quantitative Studies* (Princeton, 1975), pp. 83–98; H. M. Feinberg, "New Data on European Mortality in West Africa: The Dutch on the Gold Coast, 1719–1760," *Journal of African History*, XV (1974), 357–71.

11. P. Labarthe, *Voyage à la côte de Guinée* (Paris, 1805), p. 182.

12. Tom W. Shick, "A Quantitative Analysis of Liberian Colonization from 1820 to 1843 with Special Reference to Mortality," *Journal of African History*,

XII (1971), 45–59; John Peterson, *Province of Freedom: A History of Sierra Leone, 1787–1870* (London, 1969), pp. 28–30.

13. Al-Bakri, on ancient Ghana, cited in J. Spencer Trimingham, *A History of Islam in West Africa* (London, 1962), p. 54.

14. Philip D. Curtin, "Epidemiology and the Slave Trade," *Political Science Quarterly*, LXXXIII (1968), 190–216; Philip D. Curtin, *Economic Change in PreColonial Africa: Senegambia in the Era of the Slave Trade* (Madison, 1975), pp. 177–78; Alfred W. Crosby, "Virgin Soil Epidemics as a Factor in the Aboriginal Depopulation in America," *The William and Mary Quarterly*, XXXIII (1976), 289–99. J. F. E. Bloss surveyed the early literature for references to disease in one country and discussed the results in "Notes on the Health of the Sudan Prior to the Present Government," *Sudan Notes and Records*, XXIV (1941), 131–43.

15. G. M. Theal, *Ethnography and Condition of South Africa Before 1505* (London, 1910), p. 397; C. W. Dixon, *Smallpox* (London, 1962), p. 208.

16. See, for example, the chapter by James W. Brown in this volume.

17. Willem Bosman, *A New and Accurate Description of the Coast of Guinea* (1705; reprinted London, 1967), p. 108; K. David Patterson, "The Vanishing Mpongwe: European Contact and Demographic Change in the Gabon River," *Journal of African History*, XVI (1975), 227–28; Eugenia W. Herbert, "Smallpox Innoculation in Africa," *Journal of African History*, XVI (1975), 539–59.

18. R. Hoeppli, *Parasitic Disease in Africa and the Western Hemisphere: Early Documentation and Transmission by the Slave Trade* (Acta Tropica, suppl. 10, Basel, 1969); Sherburne F. Cook and Woodrow Borah, *Essays in Population History: Mexico and the Caribbean* (Berkeley, 1971).

19. The important role of several diseases introduced from Africa is described in John Duffy, *Epidemics in Colonial America* (Baton Rouge, 1953, 1971), *passim;* and a study of one colony is available in Peter H. Wood, *Black Majority: Negroes in Colonial South Carolina from 1670 through the Stono Rebellion* (New York, 1974). The topic deserves further attention.

20. Depopulation during the nineteenth century has been noted among the Maasai, Haya, and Kerebe; see Harry Johnston, *The Uganda Protectorate* (New York, 1904), II, 828–29; A. Arkell-Hardwick, *An Ivory Trader in North Kenia* (London, 1903), p. 232; Gerald W. Hartwig, *The Art of Survival in East Africa: The Kerebe and Long-Distance Trade, 1800–1895* (New York, 1976), pp. 122–23, 129–34, 186–88.

21. James Christie, *Cholera Epidemics in East Africa* (London, 1876).

22. See Gerald W. Hartwig, "Economic Consequences of Long-Distance Trade in East Africa: The Disease Factor," *African Studies Review*, XVIII (1975), 63–73; Aylward Shorter, *Chiefship in Western Tanzania: A Political History of the Kimbu* (Oxford, 1972), p. 39.

23. Sherman A. James and David G. Kleinbaum, "Socioecologic Stress and Hypertension Related Mortality Rates in North Carolina," *American Journal of Public Health*, LXVI, 4 (1976), 354–58; John Cassel, "The Contribution of the Social Environment to Host Resistance," *American Journal of Epidemiology*, CIV, 2 (1976), 107–23.

24. C. Van Onselen, "Reactions to Rinderpest in Southern Africa, 1896–1897," *Journal of African History*, XIII (1972), 473–88.

25. See, for example, Sèkéné-Mody Cissoko, "Famines et épidémies à Tombouctou et dans la Boucle du Niger du XVIe au XVIIIe siècle," *Bulletin de l'Institut Fondamental d'Afrique Noire*, sér. B., XXX (1968), 806–21. Bosman's *New and Accurate Description* and other accounts of the West African coast sometimes mention diseases like smallpox and syphilis.

26. K. David Patterson, "Vanishing Mpongwe"; Hartwig, the chapter on social consequences of disease in this volume, and in "Changing Forms of Servitude Among the Kerebe (Tanzania)," in *Slavery in Africa,* Suzanne Miers and Igor Kopytoff, eds. (Madison, 1977), pp. 274–83. North American Indians sometimes tried to replace lost kinsmen by adopting white captives. James Axtell, "The White Indians of Colonial America," *The William and Mary Quarterly,* XXXII (1975), 55–88.

27. Hartwig, *The Art of Survival,* pp. 182–201; A. J. H. Latham, "Witchcraft Accusations and Economic Tension in Pre-Colonial Old Calabar," *Journal of African History,* XIII (1972), 349–60.

28. K. David Patterson, "The Influenza Epidemic of 1918–19 in the Gold Coast," to appear in *Transactions of the Historical Society of Ghana;* Diana Ellis, "The Nandi Protest of 1923 in the Context of African Resistance to Colonial Rule in Kenya," *Journal of African History,* XVII (1976), 526.

29. B. B. Waddy, "African Epidemic Cerebro-Spinal Meningitis," *Journal of Tropical Medicine and Hygiene,* LX (1957), 179–89, 218–23.

30. For trypanosomiasis, see John Ford, *The Role of the Trypanosomiases in African Ecology: A Study of the Tsetse Fly Problem* (Oxford, 1971).

31. A. W. Cardinall, *The Gold Coast, 1931* (Accra, 1932), p. 220; C. W. De Kiewiet, *A History of South Africa: Social and Economic* (London, 1941), pp. 160–62; Sidney Kark and Guy Stuart, eds., *A Practice of Social Medicine: A South African Team's Experiences in Different African Communities* (Edinburgh, 1962), pp. 194–96; Isaac Schapera, *Migrant Labor and Tribal Life* (New York, 1947), pp. 156, 174–77. For an example of health conditions in one mining area, see Charles Perrings, " 'Good Lawyers' but Poor Workers'; Recruited Angolan Labour in the Copper Mines of Katanga, 1917–1921," *Journal of African History,* XVIII (1977), 245–50.

32. Charles C. Hughes and John M. Hunter, "Disease and 'Development' in Africa," *Social Science and Medicine,* III (1970), 443–93.

33. Robert S. Desowitz, "How the Wise Men Brought Malaria to Africa," *Natural History,* LXXXV, 18 (1976), 36.

34. This idea was suggested to us by Philip Curtin at the African Studies Association meeting in Boston in November 1976. For early attempts at urban sanitation, see Raymond E. Dumett, "The Campaign Against Malaria and the Extension of Scientific Medical and Sanitary Services in British West Africa, 1898–1910," *African Historical Studies,* I (1968), 153–97. African and European urban mortality is described in Pierre Cantrelle, "Mortality: Levels, Patterns, and Trends," in Caldwell, ed., *Population Growth and Socioeconomic Change in West Africa,* pp. 117–18; and E. A. Wrigley, *Population and History* (New York, 1969), pp. 95–96, 174–75. The latter book is a superb nontechnical introduction to historical demography.

35. Thomas McKeown, R. G. Record, and R. D. Turner, "An Interpretation of the Decline of Mortality in England and Wales During the Twentieth Century," *Population Studies,* XXIX (1975), 391–422; Robert Higgs, "Mortality in Rural America, 1870–1920: Estimates and Conjectures," *Explorations in Economic History,* X (1973), 177–95. One of us (K. David Patterson) is working on this problem for the Gold Coast.

36. Charles Singer and E. A. Underwood, *A Short History of Medicine* (New York, 1962) and H. H. Scott, *A History of Tropical Medicine* (Baltimore, 1939, 2 vols.) are standard sources.

37. David Scott, *Epidemic Disease in Ghana, 1901–1960* (London, 1965), p. viii.

38. European patent medicines were extensively advertised in the African

press as, for example, in the *Gold Coast Leader* throughout the colonial period.

39. See, for example, David Kimble, *A Political History of Ghana, 1850–1928* (Oxford, 1963), pp. 97–98, 105–9.

40. Asa Briggs, "Cholera and Society in the Nineteenth Century," *Past and Present*, XIX (1961), 76–96. For an excellent example, see Charles E. Rosenberg, *The Cholera Years: The United States in 1832, 1849, and 1866* (Chicago, 1962).

41. Harvey G. Soff, "Sleeping Sickness in the Lake Victoria Region of British East Africa 1900–1915," *African Historical Studies*, II (1969), 255–68; Mario Azevedo's chapter in this volume; Catherine Coquery-Vidrovitch, *Le Congo au temps des grandes compagnies concessionnaires 1898–1930* (Paris, 1972), 494–6.

42. The chapter by K. David Patterson and Gerald W. Hartwig's chapter on relapsing fever in this volume; B. B. Waddy, "Frontiers and Disease in West Africa," *Journal of Tropical Medicine and Hygiene*, LXI (1958), 100–107.

43. The Centre of African Studies at the University of Edinburgh sponsored a seminar on African Historical Demography in April 1977. Also, see R. M. A. van Zwanenberg with Anne King, *An Economic History of Kenya and Uganda, 1800–1970* (London, 1975); chap. i examines population growth in Kenya and Uganda during the past century. Equally important is Helge Kjekshus, *Ecology Control and Economic Development in East African History; The Case of Tanganyika, 1850–1950* (Berkeley, 1977); see footnote 16, chap. ii, for a comment on this study.

44. K. David Patterson, "Disease and Medicine in African History," and bibliographical essay in this volume.

2

Social Consequences of Epidemic Diseases: The Nineteenth Century in Eastern Africa

Gerald W. Hartwig

Long-distance trade intruded upon East African societies such as the Tanzanian Kerebe for the greater part of the nineteenth century. A costly part of this experience was the repeated introduction of diseases common to Indian Ocean communities but uncommon to those in the East African interior. The reverse situation was also true: newcomers encountered a varied and hostile epidemiological environment in East Africa which also took a significant toll in energy and life. Thus, we have during the nineteenth century the gradual meshing of two formerly distinct disease environments with the people participating directly in long-distance trade acting as the agents of transmission. Some of these diseases were immediately more harmful than others. Smallpox and cholera, introduced into the East African interior during this century, represent two of the most feared epidemic diseases. East Africans of the interior had no immunity to either one and the subsequent loss of life among the victims was high. Other diseases, whether venereal or those of the digestive tract, affected the health of people over a longer period of time without necessarily causing death.

From oral evidence of the Tanzanian Kerebe three social changes emerge in conjunction with the introduction of epidemic disease: altering lineage relationships, increasing accusations of sorcery, and a desire for a servile population. These and other changes are directly related to the perception of a decreasing population which was a consequence of new epidemic diseases that accompanied long-distance trade. The fundamental question asked here of the Kerebe evidence—or of evidence from any other society—is how did epidemic diseases affect them at a particular time. If we can achieve an understanding of how demographic variables such as disease affect people's lives, then we can examine the existing data and discern how people responded to an increasingly complex and lethal disease environment. Some sort of response was essential. People do not typically remain unconcerned when deaths suddenly increase for reasons unknown. East Africans can therefore be expected to have dealt with their modified epidemiological environment in ways meaningful to them.

When examining the impact of disease upon East Africans, it is assumed that we are dealing with an indiscriminate force that affected most directly those persons and communities specifically involved in long-distance trade.[1] Unfortunately, statistics relating East African mortality to epidemic disease either do not exist or are only vague estimates. From data used thus far it is exceedingly difficult to determine whether there was depopulation or population stability or even growth during the century. Those comments preserved in print by European observers are, in fact, both impressionistic and few. They are also difficult to use, as the following examples discussing smallpox and cholera will show.

In the late 1850s the explorer Richard Burton recorded this observation among the Nyamwezi in the interior of eastern Africa:

As might be expected among a sparse population leading a comparatively simple life, the vast variety of diseases which afflict more civilized races, who are collected in narrow spaces, are unknown in East Africa, even by name. . . . The most dangerous epidemic is . . . small-pox, which . . . sweeps at times like a storm of death over the land. For years it has not left the Arab colony at Kazeh, and, shortly before the arrival of the expedition, in a single month 52 slaves died out of a total of 800. . . . The Arabs have partially introduced the practice of inoculating, anciently known in South Africa. . . . The Arab merchants of Unyanyembe [Tabora] declare that, when they first visited Kargwah [Karagwe], the people were decimated by the taun, or plague. They describe correctly the bubo under the axillae, the torturing thirst, and the rapid fatality of the disease.[2]

In this statement Burton introduces a valid principle of epidemiology, that a relatively isolated and sparse population is infected by fewer diseases than a dense population having frequent contact with other societies.[3] His comment also illustrates how ivory-seeking caravans introduced diseases, such as plague in Karagwe, wherever they traveled. Furthermore, when smallpox became endemic at Kazeh, periodic outbreaks of the disease would be the norm. The slave population thus required a constant infusion of additional people.

Other observations agree with Burton's. Two decades later Dr. E. J. Southon of the London Missionary Society recorded the following estimate: ". . . the average life of males [in Unyamwezi] does not exceed twenty to twenty-five years. Many men are every year killed in battle, and great numbers fall victim to epidemics and famines."[4] Further north, in Buganda, C. T. Wilson of the Church Missionary Society also testified to the scourge of smallpox: "one of the most fatal [diseases to which the Ganda are subject], coming at intervals in epidemics, and carrying off thousands of victims; few attacked ever recover."[5] Dr. James Christie agreed that "there is no disease in East Africa so fatal in its ravages as small-pox."[6]

James Christie compiled the most impressive body of data relating the diffusion of epidemic disease through vast expanses of eastern Africa to the passages of caravans. As a medical officer on Zanzibar during the devastating cholera epidemic of 1869–70, he traced the disease into and through the interior by systematically interviewing caravan leaders and European missionaries as well as consulting existing European reports. Eventually he mapped at least a portion of the trade routes over which cholera had been conveyed by caravans.

In Christie's view, Zanzibar, and presumably much of the East African coast, prior to the outbreak in 1869–70 had experienced three major cholera epidemics: in 1821, in 1836–37,[7] and in 1858–

59. The timing of the latter epidemic coincided with the arrival of Richard Burton's exploratory expedition. Christie cited Burton, who recorded: "We lost nearly all our crew by the cholera, which, after ravaging the eastern coast of Arabia and Africa, and the islands of Zanzibar and Pemba, had almost depopulated the southern settlements on the mainland."[8] Christie commented:

The fearful nature of the epidemic as seen by Captain Burton at Kilwa, is merely an illustration of its ravages along the whole of the Zanzibar coast, for General Rigby, who was then her Majesty's Consul and Political Agent at Zanzibar, states that many of the coast towns were almost decimated.[9]

An estimated 20,000 people died of cholera on Zanzibar within a four-month period, seven to eight thousand in and immediately around the town of Zanzibar itself.[10]

Based on a conversation in 1862 between the explorer John Speke and Kabaka Mutesa of Buganda, Christie assumed that the epidemic of 1858–59 had moved along the trade routes into the interior as far as Buganda. Speke noted, however, only that Mutesa was extremely anxious to understand the disease since it had "created much mortality." Mutesa wanted to know: "What brought the scourge? What could cure it?"[11] Mutesa, according to Speke's account, implied that cholera had erupted in Buganda on more than one occasion in the past, a significant implication in view of Christie's information and Kerebe oral evidence discussed below. Finally, Christie came to believe that there had been serious mortality in what is now eastern Kenya, specifically districts inhabited by the Maasai and Galla as well as along the coast itself: "upon these extensive districts the epidemic appeared with the greatest intensity, and the mortality was described as appalling."[12]

While these observations are suggestive, they do not provide enough information to formulate a meaningful hypothesis regarding the impact of disease upon any given community. It is clear that caravans participating in long-distance trade introduced deadly epidemic diseases to people with whom the caravans traded, but the frequency of such epidemics, the actual mortality, and the social, political, or religious effects of these epidemics

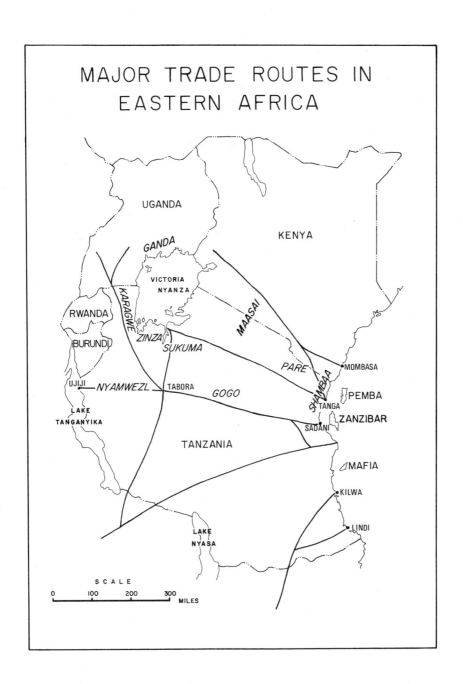

MAJOR TRADE ROUTES IN EASTERN AFRICA

UGANDA

KENYA

GANDA

VICTORIA
NYANZA

KARAGWE

MAASAI

RWANDA

BURUNDI

ZINZA

SUKUMA

PARE

MOMBASA

SHAMBAA

UJIJI NYAMWEZI TABORA GOGO

PEMBA

TANGA

LAKE
TANGANYIKA

ZANZIBAR

SADANI

TANZANIA

MAFIA

KILWA

LAKE
NYASA

LINDI

SCALE

0   100   200   300
MILES

upon the people concerned simply cannot be discerned from the evidence of these European observers. Nonetheless, it can be assumed that the loss of life among societies in periodic contact with caravans was sufficiently high and sufficiently different from anything experienced before to require a physical and psychological adjustment to a seriously altered disease environment.

Recently historians have become aware of the significance of epidemic disease. D. A. Low, for example, elaborating on Christie's impressionistic evidence, discusses the effects of both human and animal disease upon the pastoral Maasai who became unsuspecting agents of transmission for cholera in 1869 when a Maasai "raiding party contracted cholera from the Samburu." According to Low, the cholera "spread like wildfire and in a month or two was killing off large numbers" of Maasai all over their district. "It must have been the same with the extremely serious smallpox outbreak in about 1883–84, and with the pleuropneumonia which decimated their herds" later in the decade:

It was these lethal epidemics, rather than anything that occurred in war, which constituted the most serious inroads upon the strength of the 'Masai proper' at this time, and marked the first stage in their decline from their previous most formidable position.[13]

The Maasai are only one society acknowledged to have been seriously harmed by epidemic disease. West of the Victoria Nyanza in Tanzania, the kingdom of Karagwe was shattered during the 1890s by political and epidemiological factors:

The internecine wars between princes and contenders to the throne, the atrocities of the regents Kakoko and Kaketo, together with epidemics and other pestilences set Karagwe on the decline. . . . The rinderpest epidemic and the outbreak of smallpox in the early and mid-1890s reduced further the already dwindling human and animal population of Karagwe.[14]

The hypothesis that epidemic diseases depopulated East African societies toward the end of the nineteenth century seems a reasonable one, but John Iliffe has suggested the reverse, that most districts of what is now Tanzania experienced population growth during the nineteenth century. He assumes that new crops, specifically maize and rice, enabled societies to increase their numbers. "The effects of these crop changes on agricultural systems are very uncertain, but there is some evidence that they were associated with, or permitted, another nineteenth-century trend, population growth." Iliffe interprets several developments as evidence for an increasing population. His first example illustrates the nature of his evidence: "The adoption of upland rice in Matumbi seems to have been simultaneous with a growing fragmentation of clan land and an increasing number of inter-clan disputes, which suggests a growing population."[15] Other examples are similar: movement of people into previously unoccupied land implies population pressure. Immigration into the country from the south (Mozambique), east (Zaire), and north (Kenya) reinforces Iliffe's case for increased population. "Although warfare, the slave trade, and famine may have depopulated certain areas, it is likely that the country's total population grew significantly in the nineteenth century, and it is possible that this was one reason for the larger political units created in that period."[16] In Iliffe's view the devastation wrought by epidemics upon the Maasai and upon the kingdom of Karagwe would be atypical; the occupancy of vacant land was a natural expansion reflecting crowded conditions.

Yet the converse—that depopulation not population growth occurred during the nineteenth century—is more likely. "Fragmentation of clan land and an increasing number of inter-clan disputes" can be interpreted in precisely the opposite way: increased social and political tensions disrupted former relationships; therefore there was migration to ease explosive conditions. The evidence for assuming that depopulation was the critical concern of societies is stronger still if we recognize the role of epidemic disease accompanying long-distance trade. The major qualification to bear in mind is that not all East African societies actively participated in the trade. Nonetheless, the indirect consequences of that trade—whether expanding state systems, slaving activities, elephant hunting groups or disease—enveloped virtually all East Africans.

My analysis of Kerebe oral data has necessarily focused upon the probability of depopulation. Such an investigation was not my original concern, which was to reconstruct Kerebe participation in long-distance trade. But to understand that participation in its fullest sense, it became necessary to examine all leads, including a stated change in what caused people to die. This particular inquiry led to an investigation of sorcery, which in turn led to epidemic diseases.[17]

All evidence for asserting that the Kerebe experienced depopulation comes from oral sources. Two valuable contributors were Buyanza s/o Nansagate and Bahitwa s/o Lugambage.[18] Both men associated *Omukama* (Chief) Mihigo II (*ca.* 1780–*ca.* 1820) with the appearance of epidemic diseases. Bahitwa, for example, claimed that smallpox (*obulundu*) and cholera (*ensese*) arrived during the reign of Mihigo II:

[The diseases] were both supposed to have come from the Kangara [Datog]. Cholera, smallpox and tumors all came from there. I don't know where the Kangara got these diseases. Mihigo asked the Kangara to give him such diseases so he could send them to people who tried to abuse him. In this way the disease spread to all Kerebe.[19]

Buyanza conveyed the same assumption although he linked epidemic disease to sorcery:

Diseases such as cholera and smallpox were first in evidence during the rule of Mihigo II. Under Ibanda [*ca.* 1830–*ca.* 1835] people began to suspect that sorcery was being used. When diseases came and many people died, then people started to say that someone was a sorcerer because he could make a certain medicine to kill a person. Before that, people were only disturbed by fever; sucking blood out with a cow's horn could cure it. Moreover, not as many children died as today. When old men and women die, people don't mind as much as when a young person dies. Before Ibanda there were no sorcerers, drinking medicines, or taboos; these appeared when diseases came during Ibanda's time.[20]

It is not surprising that the Kerebe associate Mihigo II with the introduction of disease. He was the same *omukama* (chief) who began trading ivory for trade goods, thus initiating Kerebe participation in long-distance trade. The unusual aspect of the oral data is that it consistently links disease with the Kangara (the pastoral Datog) who inhabited an area to the east of the Kerebe. The small caravans sent by Mihigo with ivory never went to the east but always south into Sukumaland, to a place called Takama. Presumably caravans could also have returned from the south with disease. But it is not remembered that way. During the reign of Ibanda in the early 1830s, epidemic diseases became a serious problem for the community, whereas under Mihigo II neither Bahitwa nor Buyanza perceives diseases as an issue of major concern although they were present. They recall Mihigo as an all-powerful ruler, with absolute control over all aspects of life, including the disease environment. Without his sanction nothing happened, whether of a beneficial or a harmful nature. He is perceived as the last of the Kerebe *abakama* (chiefs) with this type of omnipotent authority.[21]

Mihigo's death about 1820 marks a sharp division between the old and the new. Buyanza's remarks above reflect this division. He refers to Mihigo and then to Ibanda as though the latter succeeded Mihigo in office. But Ibanda was the fourth man to hold office after Mihigo's death. The three men who preceded Ibanda all had very brief reigns: two died in office and one was deposed. Ibanda himself was also deposed after a relatively short reign for failure to end an exceedingly severe drought.[22] Thus, within about fifteen years the Kerebe experienced a great deal of political instability. Six men held office during this relatively brief interlude, with Mihigo II at the beginning of the period and his son Machunda (*ca.* 1835–*ca.* 1869) at the end. It is during this time of political turmoil that sorcery emerged as a problem. Today's elders do not consider sorcery a problem under Mihigo, because Mihigo himself is assigned responsibility for all deaths or illness attributed to epidemic diseases. All subsequent rulers "lost" control over these diseases. Yet the causation for any disease-related illnesses or deaths had to be found and it was frequently expressed in terms of sorcery, i.e., someone in the family or village was responsible. The suddenness of death common to epidemic diseases was particularly suspicious in Bahitwa's view:

Immediately after Mihigo, people began to die within a few days of the first ailments. Since people began to die when they were young,

accusations of sorcery started and all people began to condemn someone else whenever there were such misfortunes.[23]

From the beginning of the century until the late 1870s, the
Kerebe actively participated in the ivory trade. Caravans led by
Nyamwezi (or Sukuma), Arab, and Swahili traders frequented
the island community from as early as the 1830s into the 1860s.[24]
Periodic epidemics were the norm during this era, particularly
under *Omukama* Machunda (*ca.* 1835–*ca.* 1869). Because the
Kerebe had no immunity to smallpox, cholera, or other new diseases, the mortality was high. The observations and assessments
of Burton, Speke, Southon, and Christie confirm this universal
characteristic of deadly epidemic diseases.

But what oral evidence is there for depopulation? The evidence is necessarily circumstantial, since even estimates of mortality from epidemic diseases are impossible to provide. Six different conditions are mentioned by Kerebe elders that support
the assertation of depopulation. First, Mihigo II is associated in
two very distinct ways with increased deaths within the chiefdom: he "introduced" epidemic diseases and he "created" the
man/beast Butamile. Depending on the elder being questioned
about Butamile, a picture is conjured up of either a man-eating
lion or a deranged man draped in a lion skin and acting in every
way like a killer-lion. But regardless of what or who Butamile
was, it/he maimed, killed, and generally terrorized the Kerebe
for a number of years. One reason given for Mihigo's "creation"
of Butamile was that there were "too many people." A second
fact suggesting depopulation is that during the reign of Mihigo
II, the Kerebe acquired a large portion of their scarce hoe-han-
dles from Buzinza, outside the chiefdom. Wood from only two
particular species of hardwood trees possessed the required dura-
bility. Yet by mid-century it was no longer necessary to journey
to Buzinza. A sufficient supply was available within Bukerebe, a
possible consequence of reduced demand. Third, when the population of the chiefdom increased dramatically between World
War I and II, largely from immigration, and the interior of
Bukerebe had been cleared for cultivation and inhabitation, well-

used grinding stones were found in the bush, indicating that the area had been inhabited at some time in the past, allegedly during Mihigo's time. Fourth, at mid-century Machunda consciously encouraged immigration into his chiefdom, even to the extent of sending the royal canoe associated with his office to transport migrants to the island chiefdom. "Too many people" is never used after Mihigo's time to explain an *omukama's* particular course of action. Fifth, after mid-century some Kerebe actively sought to acquire and incorporate non-Kerebe children into their lineages in a servile capacity (this factor is discussed at greater length below). And sixth, the increased number of "sudden deaths" after 1830 alerts us to additional mortality even though these deaths are attributed to sorcery.

The Kerebe paid a substantial price in human life for their participation in long-distance trade. From early in the century caravans visited the chiefdom to collect ivory and thereby exposed the community repeatedly to epidemic and other diseases. From another perspective, however, the Kerebe were fortunate in that, with the exception of one devastating raid by the Baganda in 1878, they escaped serious raiding from stronger societies. But the question under consideration is not the extent of depopulation, which can only be raised not answered, but, rather, what happened to the society as a consequence of its loss?

To understand the social forces at work, we must recognize that long-distance trade was accompanied by growth in regional trade. While the *omukama* controlled long-distance exchange, his subjects dominated regional trade, mainly in grain (sorghum and millet) and in dried fish, canoes, and oars. By mid-century only one necessity—metal hoes from Buzinza—was required from outside the chiefdom. But if anyone outside the chiefdom required grain, the Kerebe would exchange it for cattle, goats, hides, hoes, or servile persons.

Except for acquiring hoes, not all Kerebe participated actively in the regional trade. Those who did were approximately one-fifth to one-fourth of the adult males. Their participation required them to produce an annual grain surplus, in the expectation that they might be able to exchange the surplus before the next harvest. To acquire possessions—whether livestock, hoes, or servile children—became their objective. Their wealth was used to improve their social position since it enabled them to become *enfura,* friends of the *omukama.* These *enfura* were the "new men" of Kerebe society. Their activities revolved around the personality in office who, in turn, depended upon them for political support. If a man could achieve the unofficial status of *enfura,* he was as secure as anyone within the chiefdom could be. The *enfura,* it should be stressed, are consistently referred to as individuals, not as members of a particular lineage. Hence, the economic and social endeavors of the *enfura* illustrate the first important change, that of communal interests subordinated to individual interests.[25] This change also reflects a conscious attempt to improve one's social and economic position. Through regional economic activities, these striving men steadfastly pursued and, in some cases, achieved success: the *omukama* recognized them as *enfura.*

Simultaneously, these individuals were highly sensitive to—and no doubt indirectly exacerbated—the emerging phenomenon of sorcery, a second change. In an African context sorcery is distinguished from witchcraft in that the latter implies an unconscious responsibility for harm. The Kerebe characteristically assumed willful intent, thus it is referred to as sorcery. According to the informants Bahitwa and Buyanza, sorcery flourished after Mihigo's death early in the century because too many younger people died following brief illnesses. That the deaths may have been a consequence of cholera or smallpox was immaterial; the agent causing the disease was the important factor. A human rather than a spiritual agent was frequently blamed for having made a person sick. Mihigo's supposed introduction of diseases is a good example, though not a case of sorcery because the human agent, Mihigo, was known. Later *abakama* did not assume this responsibility, or else the Kerebe simply did not assign it to them. Instead they assumed that the responsibility rested with other persons in the society.

We now understand sorcery and witchcraft as symptoms of a society experiencing unusually great social tension. People typically prefer to seek the source of their misfortunes and upheavals within their own ranks, not within external forces or people. They prefer not to look for explanations in the spiritual realm where misfortune could be attributed to the will of God or to a disturbed ancestral spirit. Thus the Kerebe looked to their own people for the cause of a specific affliction, and apparently they found what they sought: a person who had shown ill-will toward the afflicted or had simply acted in a hostile manner toward the person who was later victimized. In turn, such attributions of sorcery were encouraged by discontent within the society, a discontent which was certainly a product of the political, economic, and social changes of the century. The *enfura,* or those who aspired to be *enfura,* had necessarily restricted their obligations to fellow lineage members; otherwise they could never have accumulated possessions, because, according to former standards, lineage elders controlled the material wealth of a lineage, and under the modified system of the nineteenth century, these elders accumulated wealth for their own purposes. As a result, expectations of others less fortunate could not always be met, a situation which fostered ill-will.

This perceptible shift from spirit-caused to man-caused responsibility for misfortune was accelerated by the presence of epidemic diseases. Although diseases did not have to be present for a belief in sorcery to evolve as it did, when disease did appear in a context of social tension as it did for the Kerebe, the consequences were frequently traumatic and tragic.

Another change—moving from a reliance upon natural increase through marriage and births to the social device of servitude for augmenting lineage membership—is also directly related to the presence of disease and to depopulation.[26] The Kerebe institution of servitude was by no means new in the nineteenth century; it dates back to at least the seventeenth. What altered dramatically was who became a servile person[27] and for what reasons. Essentially, before 1800 the state of servitude can be described as either a welfare or a penal institution. During the nineteenth century other reasons for persons entering this state were apparent: "convicted" sorcerers, accused sorcerers, gifts from other rulers, or persons acquired through the exchange of goods, e.g., grain for a child. It is clear that servile persons became an integral part of the regional trading pattern. Whereas prior to 1800 there had been no apparent effort to go outside the chiefdom to seek persons to place in servitude (the normal practice being to exchange grain for a child if starving persons came to the chiefdom specifically for that purpose), in the later period some Kerebe began to search actively for youngsters to acquire during periods of famine in neighboring districts, either by exchanging grain for them or by kidnapping them outright.

The *enfura* were among those seeking servile persons outside the chiefdom; they had the surplus grain to exchange for them and the necessary food to feed them once they were acquired. Servile persons were desired for their short-term labor potential —to help cultivate the increased amount of grain being produced. But the *enfura* hoped in the long term to incorporate them into the lineage itself. For a servile man, this occurred after two or three generations, while a woman who bore the child of a freeman became his legal wife, her child being classified as freeborn. The redemption of servile persons had also characterized early Kerebe servitude, but it decreased during the nineteenth century as children rather than adults became more and more prevalent in the newly acquired servile population.

Thus, while *Omukama* Machunda sought immigrants to people his chiefdom, some of his subjects sought to increase their own nuclear families by bringing in servile children. Their immediate value as laborers cannot be disparaged and neither can the long-term effect of adding members to a family unit. It was one means of neutralizing the effects of epidemic diseases.

It is unrealistic to generalize too boldly about the impact upon East Africans of disease or trade goods or European guns during the nineteenth century. Not all societies experienced the same phenomena. The intensity of interaction was not always the same and neither was the timing. Certainly the frequency of epidemics affected the manner in which a society related to them, just as the extent of mortality would affect societal adjustments. In addition, some societies actively pursued a militaristic course during the latter part of the century; others experienced frequent raiding. In general, violence increased in the latter part of the century as compared to the earlier decades.

It is unfortunate that historical studies published within the past decade provide little information about social and economic developments.[28] European observers of the late nineteenth century provide us with hardly more enlightenment. Rwanda is a good example. René Lemarchand states that the rulers of Rwanda lived in "a state of splendid isolation" until the colonial era, "owing as much to the natural bulwark of swamps and mountains as to the fearsome reputation they had earned among their neighbors."[29] During the 1870s the explorer H. M. Stanley learned from Ahmed bin Ibrahim, an Arab trader, that Arabs had tried on five different occasions to initiate caravan trade with Rwanda, but each time they had been prevented by the rulers of Rwanda.[30] Ahmed bin Ibrahim informed Stanley that "the Wanya-Ruanda are wicked; and because something happened when Wangwana [freemen, people we now identify as Swahili] first tried to go there, they never tolerate strangers."[31] Stanley, in a letter to the New York *Herald*, gave additional background to explain Rwanda's reluctance to trade with caravans from the coast. While not mentioning disease explicitly, it was very likely a factor in view of Richard Burton's report that the people of Karagwe "were decimated" by plague when the first Arab merchants arrived. Stanley wrote: "from this excessive love for their cattle springs their hostility which arises from a dread of evil or fear of danger. By maintaining a strict quarantine and a system of exclusiveness they hope to ward off all evil and sudden disaster to their cattle. . . ."[32]

Secondary works are more likely to support the first change discussed for the Kerebe, the increasing importance of individual interests at the expense of lineage or communal interests. C. F. Holmes and Ralph Austen characterize economic change among some Sukuma thus: "Certain individuals concentrated on the procurement of articles for trade." The satisfaction of their acquisitive urges was at the expense "of previous traditional agricultural pursuits."[33] Not unexpectedly the former economic and social stability was damaged. Perhaps even more revealing is how the authors characterize Sukuma communities in backwater areas not participating directly in long-distance trade: "[those] systems remained far more stable throughout this tumultuous period and their lives were far less complicated. . . ."[34] Rapid change and therefore social tension were simply of less concern.

Among the Pare, Isaria Kimambo collected considerable oral data suggesting that substantial changes occurred during the nineteenth century. In the political realm, Kimambo provides explicit information. Discussing Mashombo of Mshewa, a new type of successful Pare ruler, Kimambo contrasts Mashombo's source of authority ("magical" power combined with military assistance, both brought in from Taita) to that of a traditional royal clan: "But the fact is that the powers of the traditional rituals of the Wambaga clan were no longer sufficient to meet the changing organization of the society."[35] Mashombo's case is an excellent example of the altering nature of political authority; it changes from an authority based on ritual to one based on military power, that is, from a passive to an active confrontation of new situations.[36] Although Kimambo does not claim that sorcery/witchcraft increased during the nineteenth century, he indicates that Mashombo used a different method for detecting "witches": "[His] method differed from the traditional method in that it was a response to a widespread difficulty, the difficulty of a wide breakdown of order and discipline in society."[37] Interestingly, Mashombo's way of rehabilitating all those "witches" was to bring them to his place of residence where their abilities were redirected; that is, they formed his "private army."[38] Presumably a process similar to that operating within Kerebe society was also present in Pare society: increasingly misfortune was perceived as being caused by a human rather than by a spirit. The Pare, like the Kerebe, had participated in long-distance trade from the beginning of the century, particularly in supplying provisions, and thereby had exposed themselves to epidemic diseases.

A related phenomenon among both the Pare[39] and the Shambaa was the growth of spirit-possession diseases. Steven Feierman states that "the spirit-possession diseases were pathological results of the expansion of the scale of communications."[40] The Shambaa "were disturbed to the point of personal illness by the rapidity of social change."[41] Both societies were victimized by raids for slaves during the latter decades of the century. Hence the extent of fear and distrust within the community itself would be greater among them than among the Kerebe. In such an atmosphere accusations of sorcery or witchcraft could only flourish.

The Kerebe, like the Ganda, Nyamwezi, and Gogo, acquired servile people primarily for domestic purposes, although the Ganda did export up to 1,000 slaves a year in the late 1880s. Because these importing societies participated in long-distance trade and were consequently exposed to epidemic diseases on a significant scale, it seems probable that societies importing servile persons were all involved in augmenting lineage membership through the institution of servitude. Disease and other conditions that extracted a toll in human life would naturally encourage some lineage heads to do all in their power to maintain their numbers by incorporating servile individuals into their lineages. The evidence suggests that the practice was a common one.

There is not much trustworthy information about the extent of epidemic diseases in the East African interior during the nineteenth century. And evidence for their manifold social, political, religious, and economic consequences is generally available only from oral sources. Yet it is possible to ascertain from the literature of the nineteenth century vivid impressions concerning the seriousness of cholera and smallpox epidemics. These impressions serve to indicate possible directions for us to pursue. Whether, for example, depopulation was a factor for societies repeatedly exposed to epidemic disease, or whether population growth was the norm, requires examination by persons who have collected oral historical data or who will be doing so in the near future. A concerted effort to investigate an issue such as depopulation will help us understand the nature of adjustment required of East Africans during the century. Although statistics will always elude us, we can go far to gain an appreciation of the multiple implications behind long-distance trade.

That we should be endeavoring to identify social, political, economic, and religious change might appear to be self-evident. Yet precious little has been accomplished thus far for the nine-teenth century in East Africa. The major exception is found in the sphere of political change. When examining the literature on social, economic, or religious changes among East Africans we confront a virtual vacuum.[42] Altering lineage relationships, in-creasing accusations of sorcery, and a desire for a servile popula-tion—the three social changes discussed above—are good exam-ples. At this time it is very difficult to determine whether these same changes occurred in other societies. Recently published literature has focused upon other concerns. The implications of the social changes experienced by the Kerebe for other societies in East Africa are basically speculative. If sufficient evidence from other societies in fact exists, as I suspect it does, then it is mainly a matter of marshaling the information.

The complex implications of long-distance trade are gradually being recognized, but the complexity of this phenomenon has tended to overwhelm us. The political consequences alone occu-pied historians for almost a decade. Current interest is now focused upon economic questions concerning the entire society, not simply the political elite. But as significant as this latter de-velopment is, it may very well overlook equally significant social questions by taking a less than holistic approach. We can be only partially informed by asking restricting questions.

A fundamental restriction historians have imposed upon them-selves is that of considering primarily the opportunity factor as-sociated with long-distance trade, and excluding all too often the cost factor. The opportunity factor consists of determining the manner by which East Africans took advantage of altering po-litical and economic conditions associated with the trade. Yet at the same time as long-distance trade increased, those in political positions experienced considerable instability, a condition en-couraging the breakup of former political units on the one hand and the formation of larger political units on the other. Although such political instability was certainly one of the "costs," ignoring the cost factor in its other aspects has meant dismissing from consideration something as basic as epidemic disease. Therefore, the probability of depopulation, except that related to slave raiding, has not emerged as a research priority. Until the basic question of depopulation is clarified, not only will the social implications of long-distance trade be poorly understood, political and economic developments will also be inadequately assessed.

An analysis of the cost factor of long-distance trade makes the social changes at work among the Kerebe more comprehensible. Altering lineage relationships, increasing accusations of sorcery, and desire for a servile population generally connote in our minds the image of an unsavory society. But when it is acknowledged that the society was experiencing depopulation, these same social developments are perceived in a different light. The game of life is played with a different set of rules when survival is at stake.

Notes

1. The specific relationship of disease to economic factors is discussed in "Economic Consequences of Long-Distance Trade in East Africa: The Disease Factor," *African Studies Review*, XVIII, 2 (1975), 63–73.

2. Richard F. Burton, *The Lake Regions of Central Africa* (New York, 1860), p. 485. Additional information on smallpox inoculation is found in Eugenia W. Herbert, "Smallpox Inoculation in Africa," *Journal of African History*, XVI, 4 (1975), 539–60.

3. Francis L. Black recently made a related assertion: "The spectrum of diseases that afflicted man through most of his development [from Neolithic times to the present] may have been much smaller than that to which we have been subject in historic times." See "Infectious Diseases in Primitive Societies," *Science*, CLXXXVII (February 1975), 515.

4. E. J. Southon, "History, Country, and People of the Unyamwezi District," 1880, Central Africa, London Missionary Society Archives, London.

5. C. T. Wilson and Robert Felkin, *Uganda and the Egyptian Soudan* (London, 1882), I, 183.

6. James Christie, *Cholera Epidemics in East Africa* (London, 1876), p. 253.

7. *Ibid.*, 100–101. Also see Robert F. Stock, *Cholera in Africa: Diffusion of the Disease, 1970–1975, with Particular Emphasis on West Africa* (London, 1976), pp. 14–21.

8. *Ibid.*, p. 113.

9. *Ibid.*, p. 115.

10. *Ibid.*, p. 117.

11. *Ibid.*, p. 116, also pp. 106–7.

12. *Ibid.*, p. 234.

13. D. A. Low, "The Northern Interior, 1840–84," *History of East Africa*, ed. Roland Oliver and Gervase Mathew (Oxford, 1963), I, 308.

14. Israel K. Katoke, "The Making of the Karagwe Kingdom," Historical Association of Tanzania Paper No. 8 (Nairobi, 1970), p. 29; Katoke, *The Karagwe Kingdom* (Nairobi, 1975), pp. 113, 135–36.

15. John Iliffe, "Agricultural Change in Modern Tanganyika," Historical Association of Tanzania Paper No. 10 (Nairobi, 1971), p. 9.

16. *Ibid.* Two recent works have convincingly claimed that the period between 1890 and about 1925 was a time of depopulation in East Africa: R. M. A. van Zwanenberg with Anne King, *An Economic History of Kenya and Uganda, 1800–1970* (London, 1975); and Helge Kjekshus, *Ecology Control and Economic Development in East African History, The Case of Tanganyika, 1850–1950* (Berkeley, 1977). Kjekshus, in particular, supports the proposition that there was at least population stability if not growth before 1890, thereby supporting Iliffe's interpretation. On the other hand, I place greater significance on the detrimental effects of widespread droughts, and subsequent famines, and epidemic disease than does Kjekshus or Iliffe. Until more oral evidence is acquired, we can only offer interpretations because the evidence is so very meager at present.

17. See Gerald W. Hartwig, "Long-Distance Trade and the Evolution of Sorcery among the Kerebe," *African Historical Studies,* IV, 3 (1971), 505–24; and Hartwig, *The Art of Survival in East Africa: The Kerebe and Long-Distance Trade, 1800–1895* (New York, 1976), pp. 74–78, 182–204.

18. Other elders who contributed information on this subject include Alipyo Mnyaga, Aniceti Kitereza, Daudi Musombwa, Magoma s/o Kitina, Palapala s/o Kazwegulu, and Simeo Rubuzi. Information about these men can be found in *The Art of Survival in East Africa*, pp. 212–20.

19. Bahitwa s/o Lugambage, interview 28 November 1968.

20. Buyanza s/o Nansagate, interview 12 November 1968.

21. The oral data describing affairs of the nineteenth century vary from one elder to another. An established oral tradition that is repeated consistently by a number of informants does not exist around any one topic pertaining to the nineteenth century with the sole exception of the power and authority attributed to Mihigo II. But that is not really a tradition; it is a brief statement of "fact." All other remembered details about Mihigo's reign again vary significantly from elder to elder. See Hartwig, "Oral Data and Its Historical Function in East Africa," *International Journal of African Historical Studies,* VII, 3 (1974), 468–79.

22. This drought was apparently widespread in eastern Africa. Ethiopian records refer to the same time as a period of drought and famine: Richard Pankhurst, *Economic History of Ethiopia, 1800–1935* (Addis Ababa, 1968), pp. 216–17. The Kamba of Kenya suffered similarly at this time: J. L. Krapf, *Travel, Researches and Missionary Labours During an Eighteen Year's Residence in Eastern Africa* (London, 1860), p. 142.

23. Bahitwa s/o Lugambage, interview 4 February 1969.

24. See Richard Burton, *The Lake Regions of Central Africa,* pp. 415–16.

25. Andrew Roberts has identified two changes that were operative in the political sphere during the nineteenth century in eastern Africa: the development of military and economic power at the expense of ritual power as a basis for leadership, and the related emphasis on personal achievement and loyalty rather than kinship as a qualification for political office; *Tanzania Before 1900* (Nairobi, 1968), p. 15. The Kerebe experienced these changes as well as one identified by Steven Feierman that refers to a change in the perception of the most desirable form of wealth, from livestock and the labor of subjects to imported trade goods. When the latter became more important to chiefs and their advisers, subjects in turn became less important, even expendable; *The Shambaa Kingdom* (Madison, 1974), pp. 172–79.

26. Servitude among the Kerebe has been discussed at length in Hartwig, "Changing Forms of Servitude among the Kerebe of Tanzania," in *Slavery in Africa: Historical and Anthropological Perspectives,* ed. Suzanne Miers and Igor

Kopytoff (Madison, 1977), pp. 261–85; also in *The Art of Survival in East Africa*, pp. 103–39.

27. I use 'servile person' in preference to 'slave' because of cultural connotations attached to the word *slave*. Servitude in most African societies was markedly different from chattel slavery. When a person was destined for the international slave market, then the word *slave* is used; the person is then a commodity. Suzanne Miers and Igor Kopytoff provide an excellent discussion of terminology in *Slavery in Africa*, pp. 3–7.

28. My colleague, John W. Cell, makes this assessment about oral historians: "There is a paradox here. African historians have been extremely innovative in pioneering the use of oral evidence. But they have been conservative in selecting the topics they chose to investigate." Personal communication, 30 March 1977.

29. René Lemarchand, *Rwanda and Burundi* (New York, 1970), p. 47.

30. Norman R. Bennett, ed., *Stanley's Despatches to the New York Herald, 1871–1872, 1874–1877* (Boston, 1970), p. 273.

31. Henry M. Stanley, *Through the Dark Continent* (London, 1899 edition), I, 368.

32. Bennett, *Stanley's Despatches to the New York Herald*, p. 280.

33. C. F. Holmes and R. A. Austen, "The Pre-Colonial Sukuma," *Journal of World History*, XIV, 2 (1972), 392.

34. *Ibid.*, p. 396.

35. Isaria N. Kimambo, *A Political History of the Pare of Tanzania, c. 1500–1900* (Nairobi, 1969), p. 149.

36. See footnote 25 above regarding political changes.

37. Kimambo, *History of the Pare*, p. 151.

38. *Ibid.* Changing social roles are also discussed by Kennell Jackson, "The Dimensions of Kamba Pre-Colonial History," *Kenya Before 1900: Eight Regional Studies*, ed. B. A. Ogot (Nairobi, 1976), pp. 176–78, 238.

39. *Ibid.*, pp. 189–90.

40 Feierman, *The Shambaa Kingdom*, p. 201.

41. *Ibid.*, p. 202.

42. The Kjekshus volume, *Ecology Control and Economic Development in East African History*, is explicitly a book of protest. The author, a political scientist, was sufficiently frustrated by the narrowness of historical works to venture into the arena himself and write a more holistic, comprehensive type of history, one that would be more beneficial to nonspecialists.

3

Man, Milieu, and the Disease Factor: Tick-Borne Relapsing Fever in East Africa

Charles M. Good

Tropical Africa has long held a well-deserved reputation as a vast breeding ground and dispersal center for dozens of diseases that variously debilitate or decimate human and domestic animal populations. Nevertheless, the pervasiveness and systematic interplay of the disease factor in African life has received little analysis or interpretation in assessments of the colonial era. This critical oversight may have been reinforced by a popular but uninformed belief that disease is a problem of the "natural" environment, and thus is unrelated to questions of social, cultural, and economic change. Neglect of the disease factor has undoubtedly also been partly due to the notion that disease is too complex and mysterious for social scientists and historians who lack a medical degree or other specialist training in the life sciences to consider intelligently. Fortunately, the traditional compartmentalization and narrow definition of disciplinary boundaries is gradually giving way to a recognition of the merits of holism and greater interdisciplinary communication.[1] More than ever before, we are challenged not to concoct deterministic explanations of societal change in terms of disease, but to strive for a more balanced evaluation of the African experience by clarifying when, where, how, and why disease has been significant.

In this chapter, I focus on the relationship of tick-borne relapsing fever to the changing patterns of human activity, human organization, and man-environment interactions in the interior of East Africa generally, and Uganda in particular. My historical frame of reference is the late nineteenth century and the brief but momentous colonial period which followed. For the Africans who were invaded, the period beginning with the late 1870s featured unprecedented contact with alien cultures and participation in processes, both direct and subtle, which would soon transform indigenous concepts of time and space. The rise and diffusion of relapsing fever is a product of these extraordinary circumstances. Although relapsing fever is typically a disease of low mortality and has seldom challenged the established dominance of other vector-borne parasitic diseases such as malaria and trypanosomiasis, it has constituted a serious public health problem in extensive areas of East Africa. Now that the disease appears to have entered a quiescent period across most of the region, it seems appropriate, despite deficiencies in statistical data, to chart its course and begin evaluating its relationship to the colonial systems and environments of East Africa.

Relapsing Fever: Status and General Characteristics

Two forms of relapsing fever occur in Africa. *Louse*-borne relapsing fever, transmitted by anthropophilic *Pediculus humanus*, is confined to a few areas including Ethiopia, Sudan, and Zaire (see chapter 8). In 1969, 90 percent of the 5,117 cases reported to the World Health Organization occurred in Ethiopia, "the only known definite endemic focus of the disease existing in the world today."[2] *Tick*-borne relapsing fever is endemic in discontinuous but extensive areas of eastern, south central, and southeastern Africa. In recent years, cases have been reported from Chad, Angola, Malawi, Rwanda, Burundi, Uganda, and Kenya. There is also reason to suspect, on the basis of previous experience of the disease, that several other countries should be represented in the list but have chosen not to notify the international agency. Countries outside of Africa reporting cases of tick-borne relapsing fever since 1966 include Colombia, Jordan, Israel, Pakistan, Portugal, Spain, and Kuwait.[3]

David Livingstone was perhaps the first to note a possible relationship between tick-bite and fever after having been bitten in

1857 by a "Tampan" tick at Ambaca in northwest Angola.[4] Other observers, including Sir John Kirk, and S. L. Hinde, who led an expedition to the Congo Free State in 1892–94, reported a similar disease in the Zambezi Valley and eastern Congo.[5] In 1904, the researches of A. R. Cook[6] and P. H. Ross and A. D. Milne[7] in Uganda, and those of J. E. Dutton and J. L. Todd[8] working independently in the Congo Free State, demonstrated that the causative agent of relapsing fever is a spirochete or spiral bacterium, _Borrelia duttoni_, carried in the blood of infected persons. The most common vector of this pathogen is the domestic tick _Ornithodorus moubata_[9] or its progeny (there is transovarial transmission) which have previously bitten an infected person. This tick does not usually travel more than thirty yards by itself and is thus dependent on man or animals for transport to other locations.[10] It inhabits cracks and crevices in the walls and mud floors of African dwellings, resthouses, hoteli, and campsites along trade and migratory labor routes, and it may infest urban rented quarters, schools, and prisons. Most East African peoples reportedly recognize _O. moubata_ and the disease it causes.[11]

The consequences of relapsing fever in East Africa in terms of human mental and physical health and socioeconomic development remain to be systematically identified. Although local immunity tends to mask the extent of morbidity, the disease can be severe and disabling. Clinically, relapsing fever is characterized at the onset by a high fever and, commonly, diarrhea and dysenteric symptoms. Apyrexial intervals are irregular and may last from one day to three weeks. Up to eleven relapses may occur, with accompanying cerebral complications and possible optic atrophy. The patient's liver and spleen are usually enlarged, and jaundice, bronchitis, and pneumonia frequently occur.[12] Circumstantial evidence of a high incidence of stillbirths in infected African women has been reported from Tanzania. Children under sixteen years of age who are still in the process of acquiring immunity are likely to contract the disease. Among diagnosed hospital cases of tick-borne relapsing fever, the mortality rate is approximately 2 percent. Maintenance of immunity in adults is thought to reduce strength critically. Moreover, ticks, together with mosquitoes, bedbugs, fleas, and other pests which invade many African dwellings, can produce night-long torture for the human occupants and may even force them to sleep outdoors, where they come in contact with other health hazards. Indeed, in terms of hindering economic development, lack of sleep because of tick molestation may be as important as the infection itself.[13]

Walton writes that the effect of relapsing fever on Africans who have no immunity to it "may be as severe as that produced by malignant tertian malaria. . . ."[14] He recounts the story of some Maasai who had been imprisoned in jail in Mwanza, Tanganyika and had died after contracting the disease. The prison may not have been infested with ticks, but most of the occupants were local Sukuma who could have brought them on their clothing. Hence, in Walton's rather scornful view, "a three months prison sentence could be three months rest with free food for the local tick-infested Sukuma tribesman and a sentence of death for the tick-free Masai who have no immunity to the disease."[15]

The entomologist Gerald Walton has a perceptive grasp of the scope of man-environment interactions and the role of culture as these bear upon disease ecology. Any assessment of the ecosystemic features and historical medical geography of tick-borne relapsing fever in eastern Africa must draw extensively on the results of his twelve years of field investigations. One important factor which his research highlights is "the probable enormous extent" of the domestic distribution of *O. moubata* in Africa south of the Sahara. In Tanzania alone, "vast and often almost continuous spatial distributions" of the tick have been discovered in human dwellings, of which one million were estimated to be infested in 1964.[16] Other areas in which the tick (and in many cases the disease) was identified during the colonial era include almost all of south central and southern Africa (except Lesotho); the remainder of East Africa, and eastern and southern Zaire; and parts of northeast Africa, including the southern Sudan and Somalia. In the latter country, the high mobility of nomadic populations undoubtedly fostered easy and rapid circulation of the tick vector. Relapsing fever became focused in the houses,

coffee shops, and other public places in the towns; colonial officials even burned down some towns in unsuccessful efforts to
control the disease.[17]

O. moubata, rather than being a single domestic species, may
be two distinct species of tick which long ago originated as ecto-
parasites of wild, burrowing animals such as the porcupine and
warthog. Although both are associated with human habitations,
they probably continue to be derived from foci in the bush.
These extremely hardy ticks have markedly different microcli-
matic preferences as well as high starvation resistance, a factor
which is significant in epidemiology and vector control. Figure 1
shows the source locations, relative to the distribution of annual
rainfall, of persons who contracted relapsing fever and were admitted to hospitals in Uganda, Kenya, and Tanganyika. Admissions came from all rainfall zones, and there are discontinuous
but extensive areas of each country in which immunity is obviously quite low.

Depending on their specific ecologic requirements and local
adaptations to domestic environments, the ticks also exhibit distinct preferences in choice of host. For example, in highland areas
of Kenya such as Nyeri and the Taita Hills, the ticks are dependent on low temperature and high relative humidity within very
narrow ranges of tolerance.[18] Here, man is the preferred host. In
contrast, the density of infestation in houses in the Digo district
south of Mombasa, Kenya, was six times that in the highlands.
The optimum microhabitat of these coast ticks was 26.6°C and
83 percent relative humidity in an area receiving 40 to 50 inches
of rainfall. Just south of this area rainfall increases to over 50
inches, and there is a close correspondence between greater rainfall and the absence of tick infestation in houses. However,
within the 80 square-mile zone of heavy tick infestation the preferred host was not man, but rather domestic fowls, the ticks
feeding on chickens 14 times as often as humans. Still a third
form of the vector was discovered in the dry central parts of
Tanzania, where the tick "feeds with equal facility on man or
domestic fowls."[19]

One of the most important aspects of the problem of relapsing fever is that tick-infested human habitations do not necessarily indicate the presence of the disease. This is because "the distribution of domestic *Ornithodorus* ticks differs markedly from that of tick-borne relapsing fever."[20] As in the case of the Digo district, if the tick's preferred host is other than man, the incidence of relapsing fever may be extremely low. Recorded cases might then result from infected transient persons and importation of infected ticks. In addition, another kind of quiescent "type-site" occurs when the ticks feed on human blood but cases of the disease are few because the entire human community exhibits a strong immunity to the infection. Again, cases which do appear are usually either immigrants or local children who have not yet acquired resistance to local strains of the spirochete. Walton hypothesizes that this immunity is a highly localized phenomenon which breaks down with population movements. Visitors to an area may originate in districts where relapsing fever is present but possibly masked by widespread local immunity. However, this does not confer cross-immunity to the disease after persons have been bitten away from home by *Ornithodorus* that harbor heterologous strains of spirochete. Since transmission of *B. duttoni* in established locations is commonly at hyperendemic levels, large scale population movements such as labor migration between foci lacking cross-immunity can touch off rampant epidemics.[21]

As humans we engage in innumerable practices or actions which serve to expose us to or shield us from disease hazards. Interactions which occur within self-contained societies are frequently "culture specific" in that they involve processes, relationships, and adaptations that result in human adjustment or maladjustment within a separate and distinct social system. The sum of these elements form a dynamic component of a society's *cultural ecology* which is ultimately reflected in its morbidity and mortality profiles.[22] These conditions are never static, of course, and the implications which the analysis of possible behavioral adjustments hold for human selection and disease control are far-reaching. As Alland, Hunter and Hughes, and many others have stressed, any modification of a behavioral system or ecological

Figure 1. *Distribution of Rainfall and Relapsing Fever in East Africa*

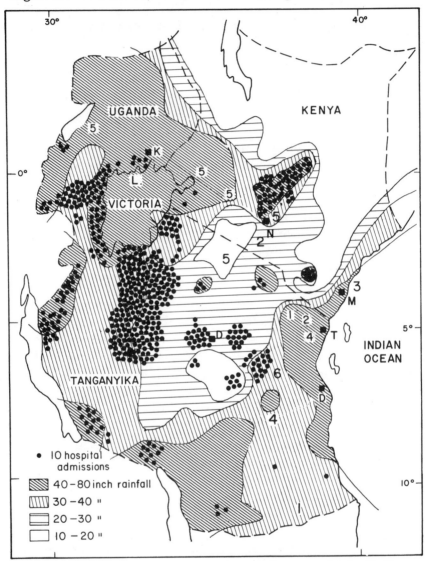

Note: D—Dar-es-Salaam; K—Kampala; M—Mombasa; N—Nairobi; T—Tanga. One dot represents 10 hospital admissions. When there were less than 10 admissions, the recorded number is shown. Thus in Kenya there were five cases in Nairobi and two in Maasailand (five on the Tanganyika side of the border). Tanganyika data are for 1952, Kenya for 1947, and Uganda for 1949. All countries were at approximately the same stage in housing development when a reduction in the incidence of infection had been established but was still high.

Source: Redrawn from G. A. Walton, *Symposium of the Zoological Society of London*, 6 (1962), 83–156, by permission of the author and the Zoological Society of London.

Figure 2. *Language and Selected Ethnic Groups in East Africa*

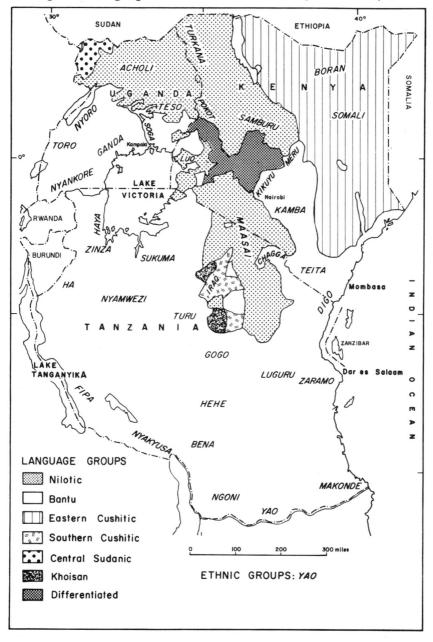

LANGUAGE GROUPS

Nilotic

Bantu

Eastern Cushitic

Southern Cushitic

Central Sudanic

Khoisan

Differentiated

ETHNIC GROUPS: *YAO*

"contract" will probably have medical consequences.[23] This concept of disease as interaction is particularly appropriate to the analysis of relapsing fever.

Fundamental differences in ethnohistory and material culture between East African pastoral and agricultural societies appear to be important in the cultural ecology of relapsing fever. A spatial association between the distribution of reported relapsing fever cases and the distribution of many Bantu-speaking groups is apparent when Figure 1 is compared with Figure 2. The general scarcity of *Ornithodorus* and relapsing fever in the northern portion of East Africa is due, Walton contends, to the occupation of the area over the past several centuries by intrusive pastoralist groups, including the Nilotic-speaking Maasai, Nandi, Kipsigis, and Luo, and the Cushitic-speaking Somali and Galla. The more nomadic and mobile of these societies construct small simple dwellings, essentially of grass, which can be as readily abandoned as they are easily built. Under these fluid conditions ticks would find it difficult to establish a domestic niche. In contrast, the more sedentary Nilotes of the pastoral tradition, such as the Luo, build round *m'songe*-type houses that have well-plastered inside walls. The women remain at the homestead, "frequently repair the plaster (a weekly routine of the Luo), keep the hut clean and free it of vermin."[24]

Among the Bantu agriculturalists, Walton theorizes that

the m'songe design was extensively copied . . . without understanding the necessity of plastering and providing an adequate integral roof support. Many interiors became cluttered with mud and wattle screens, posts to support the weak roof and strange sleeping contraptions, sleeping cells, pens for the traditional fat ram, floors were full of cracks and dusty, walls full of crevasses and the whole interior warmed, at higher altitudes, to provide ideal cover and food for ticks. Traditionally the children and in some tribes the whole family sleep on the floor. Bed platforms raised on forked posts set in the floor as an attempt to escape tick molestation are far from effective.[25]

On the other hand, the dwellings of the Bantu-speaking Kamba in Kenya are not tick infested. "Beds are raised high off the ground, and goats, tethered round the periphery, trample out tick

infestations. The people react violently to B. duttoni infection."[26]
The Bantu Sukuma who inhabit the territory stretching south of
Lake Victoria

frequently keep goats in the inner and outer circle of the traditional
dwelling. This reduces the tick infestation. After some months the
people change places with the animals. Fowls are numerous and
broody hens are kept indoors. One homestead may be infested with
ticks feeding on fowls, another with ticks which feed on man. Presumably one family may be immune and their neighbors non-immune.
Weddings, funerals and other social gatherings are followed by outbreaks of relapsing fever.[27]

Origins and Diffusion of Relapsing Fever

In 1903, Drs. J. Everett Dutton and John Todd were sent out
to the Congo Free State by the Liverpool School of Tropical
Medicine to conduct investigations of Gambian sleeping sickness.
They had frequent experiences of *Ornithodorus* and its effects
after their arrival in the Oriental province.

We found that natives who knew the arachnid had . . . a decided
dread of it; but it was not until we had left Stanleyville, on our way
up the Congo to Kasongo, that we constantly encountered the tick,
and saw, for the first time, cases of the disease. . . . We reached
Kasongo on November 23, and have here seen further cases, and have
been ourselves attacked by the disease.[28]

In February, 1905, Dutton succumbed at Kasongo to a severe
febrile disease generally assumed to be relapsing fever.[29] Before
his death he and Todd published a map showing a relationship
between the distribution of infected ticks collected or reported
in the eastern Congo and neighboring locations such as Tabora,
and the routes used by Arab caravans from the Tanganyika coast
(see Figure 3). European caravan routes in Manyema and the
Rift corridor, as well as in the lower Congo and in Portuguese
areas to the south were also suspected and mapped. Although
Dutton and Todd found a high prevalence of ticks in certain
Arabized villages in Manyema, and especially in resthouses along
the main routes, African settlements only an hour's walk away

were usually tick free. This appeared to confirm their suspicion that the rapidly expanding disease was traceable to infected ticks carried inland in the clothing and bedding of traders from the east coast.[30] However accurate this assumption may have been, it is evident that the conclusion was based upon the distribution of the tick collectors rather than the actual distribution of ticks.[31]

Also in 1905, Robert Koch's field investigations established the presence of relapsing fever on the overland route leading from the Tanganyika coast into the interior. He concluded that the disease had "always been mistaken for malaria," and had long been widely distributed and endemic in Tanganyika.

Infected ticks were found in all the locations on the caravan route from Daressalem to beyond Kilossa, in the direction of Mpapua, and on the track from Kilossa to Iringa. They were also found in the villages of the Rubeho Mountains, and in locations away from the caravan routes.[32]

These findings complemented those of Dutton and Todd. They were the basis for Koch's belief that the disease was not a recent arrival in the interior of East Africa.

Today, although the historical context is certainly better understood, knowledge of the factors which explain the rise of relapsing fever as a public health problem around the turn of the century is little more advanced than it was 60 years ago. Since the ticks are dependent upon man for transport and there is now considerable evidence that cross-immunity is localized, the implications for the disease of greater population mobility and broader networks of spatial interaction characteristic of this period are obviously quite enormous. The processes that were unleashed accelerated dispersal, relocation, mixing, and feedback of different spirochete strains in and between previously uninfected areas and old endemic zones. This integration of ticks and spirochetes considerably expanded the population at risk in many places, especially in settlements and facilities used by travelers. The routeways created by patterns of local, regional, and long-distance exchange were readily transformed into corridors of contagion, as is so perfectly illustrated by the interrelationship between the spread of sleeping sickness and the ancient system

Figure 3. *Distribution of the Human Tick, Congo Free State, 1904*

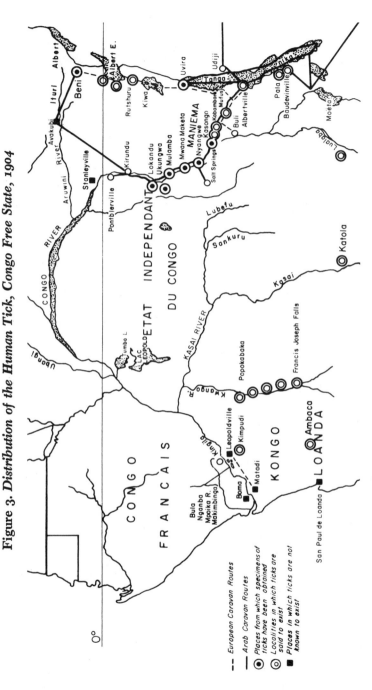

Source: Redrawn from Dutton and Todd, "The Nature of Human Tick-Fever in the Eastern Part of the Congo Free State." Liverpool School of Tropical Medicine, Memoir XVII (1905). Reprinted with permission.

of salt trading in Katwe, Kasenyi, and Kibero in the Western
Rift Valley.[33] Also hazardous to human health were military actions, movements of conscript porters and slaves, the creation of
towns and administrative posts, and compulsory resettlement of
African populations caught up in the reorganization of space by
colonial administrations.[34]

Hindle's review of relapsing fever in 1911 lists all places from
the Sudan to South Africa in which the disease had been definitely recorded (see Table 1). In his assessment, German East
Africa and the part of Uganda bordering it were then probably
"the main centre of the Relapsing Fever of Tropical Africa."[35]
The lower Zambezi valley was another important focus. From
these two centers the disease spread north and south along the
East African coast from Somalia to Zululand, from Tete into and
beyond Nyasaland via the Arab trade route along the western
side of the lake, and inland beyond Victoria Falls. Hindle accepted Dutton and Todd's findings as evidence that "the disease
has only recently been introduced into the Congo along the lines
of travel and has not yet had time to spread into the surrounding
country, as it has done in German East Africa."[36] This early assessment of the eastern Congo as a target zone rather than a
center of origin for the dissemination of relapsing fever is echoed
in a recent survey of the convergence of Western medicine and
disease in Uganda in the early twentieth century by W. D. Foster, a medical microbiologist. He suggests that relapsing fever
spread from Uganda into the Congo rather than moving in the
opposite direction like sleeping sickness and jigger fleas (*Tunga
penetrans*).[37]

Although Foster does not document his hypothesis, other evidence makes it plausible. Relapsing fever was "suspected" in
Uganda as early as 1896 by Dr. R. U. Moffat in Masindi, and
Cook actually identified the disease under the microscope in
1899.[38] As early as 1903 relapsing fever was reported from Busoga
(east of the Victoria Nile), Wadelai (on the Albert Nile), and
Katwe at Lake Edward.[39] In November of the same year Cook
reported that "a somewhat widespread epidemic seems to be

Table 1. *Early Recorded Distribution of Relapsing Fever in East Africa and Congo*

Territory	Locality	Date	Observer/ Recorder
Uganda	Masindi[1]	1896	R. U. Moffat
	Kampala (?)	1899	A. R. Cook
	Busoga	1903	Christy
	Wadelai (Nile R.)	1903	"
	Katwe (L. Edward)	1903	"
	Mbale	1907	Simpson
	Entebbe	1907	"
	Ngomanene (Buganda)	1907	"
	Lake Mamba (Buganda)	1907	"
	Mpumu Chagwe (Buganda)	1909	P. H. Ross
British East Africa	Kilimanjaro	1901	E. Brumpt
	Nairobi	1908	P. H. Ross
German East Africa	Rubeho Mts.	1905	R. Koch
	Dar-es-Salaam	1905	"
	Kilosa	1905	"
	Mpwapwa	1905	"
	Iringa	1905	"
	Tabora	1905	Dutton and Todd
Congo Free State	Kasongo	1905	Dutton and Todd
	Lokandu	1905	"
	Mulamba	1905	"
	Mwana Maketa	1905	"
	Nyangwe	1905	"
	Ukungwa	1905	"
	Uvira	1905	"
	Beni	1905	"

1. Suspected relapsing fever.
Primary source: E. Hindle, "The Relapsing Fever of Tropical Africa," 190.

raging, extending from the province of Budu in the southwest, to the borders of Kyagwe to the east" in Buganda Kingdom.[40] Shortly thereafter, it was recorded in Mbale in eastern Uganda, Entebbe, and other locations in Buganda.[41] Moffat, who was Principal Medical Officer of Uganda until 1906, saw more than 150 cases of relapsing fever during his last year in the Protectorate. He thought the disease had probably often been mistaken for malaria in the past, and was convinced it was "certainly not a new one in Uganda."[42] Neither did he doubt its increasing prevalence.

This is in great measure due to the increasing traffic on the main roads, for it is in the tick-infested camps along these roads that infection is most commonly contracted. Owing to the exigencies of food and water suitable camping grounds are only to be found at certain places and the caravans in a constant stream make use of these nightly. Once the ticks become infected it is easy to see how the disease is disseminated, and, indeed, the risk of infection is so great that it constitutes one of the most serious dangers and drawbacks to travel in Uganda at the present time.[43]

Katwe, as already noted, was a known focus of relapsing fever as early as 1903 and remained so until 1960.[44] The preexisting land and water routes of the valuable Katwe-Congo salt trade, which provided a highly efficient medium for the diffusion of sleeping sickness, quite probably also facilitated the movement of traders and ticks infected with *B. duttoni* westward and southward into the Congo. If this assumption is correct, archaeological evidence of the salt trade would put relapsing fever in the eastern Congo long before the arrival there of Coast Moslems.[45] Hence, as this review illustrates, the genesis, relative importance of difference locations, timing, and means of diffusion of the disease in the interlacustrine and Rift corridor zones remain a mystery. Similar questions remain for Kenya, where cases were first recognized in 1907. On the basis of available evidence, it appears that there were several endemic foci of relapsing fever activated during the age of exploration and early colonial administration in East and Central Africa.

Relapsing Fever in the Uganda Protectorate

Relapsing fever has recently been called a "disease of interest and importance in the medical history of Uganda."[46] It achieved this status quite early, as we have seen in the case of the epidemic which broke out in Buganda in 1903. Curiously, in 1904 there were only 33 reported cases, but in the following two years

Figure 4. Uganda and Kenya: Reported Cases of Tick-Borne Relapsing Fever, 1925–60

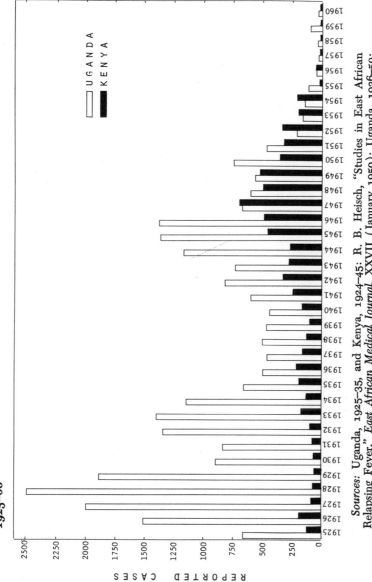

Sources: Uganda, 1925–35, and Kenya, 1924–45: R. B. Heisch, "Studies in East African Relapsing Fever," *East African Medical Journal,* XXVII (January 1950); Uganda, 1936–59: Uganda Protectorate, *Annual Report of the Medical Department,* 1960, and personal communication, Uganda Ministry of Health, 20 January 1971; Kenya, 1946–1960: E. Rodenwalt (ed.), *World Atlas of Epidemic Diseases,* II (1952); W.H.O., *Epidemiological and Vital Statistics Report,* XX, 5 (1967), 396–97; and C. Teesdale, *East African Medical Journal,* XLII (October 1965), 529–34.

there were respectively 414 and 932 cases.[47] Unfortunately, disease statistics for the period from 1907 to 1925 were not accessible although some records undoubtedly exist in the annual reports of the Principal Medical Officer housed at the Entebbe national archives. During much of this eighteen-year period, the Protectorate government was preoccupied with the ravages of sleeping sickness and its campaign against venereal diseases.[48] If the lack of references to relapsing fever in the local archives of Ankole and Kigezi Districts is an acceptable indicator, the disease remained comparatively quiescent until after World War I. However, by the mid-1920s it had reappeared in epidemic proportion and persisted as a public health threat until the mid-1950s (Figure 4). Of particular note is the special role of Buganda. It was a comparatively prosperous and labor-short region of the Protectorate when compared to its poorer labor-supplying neighbors such as Ruanda-Urundi, Tanganyika, and adjacent areas of the Congo.

Relapsing fever was apparently unknown in Kigezi District in 1920. Local British administrators attributed its introduction shortly thereafter to the pedestrian salt traffic which had long linked Katwe and Kigezi via western Ankole. By 1929, the disease was approaching epidemic scale in Kigezi, where there were estimates of considerably more than 100 deaths, including whole households.[49] Many settlements "along the main Kichwamba–Nyarushanje–Kabale–Gisolo route" had become foci of infection, as were the chiefs' town houses in Kabale, the district headquarters.[50] The district commissioner of Kigezi saw "thirteen separate cases of people in this district carrying salt who have become infected on the road (in Toro or Ankole) and were apparently dying by the roadside."[51]

If this eruption of relapsing fever in Kigezi was directly traceable to Katwe and the long-distance salt commerce, its mechanism of dispersal was soon eliminated. By 1929, the traditional organization of the salt trade was undergoing a radical change due to the introduction of motor vehicles. African foot traders were being replaced by Asian entrepreneurs who had motor lorries and could deal in wholesale quantities. The fact that pedestrian salt traders were swiftly forced out of operation because of their inability to compete with motor transportation apparently served to halt the spread of relapsing fever. In 1931, for instance, an earlier plan to construct new tick-free rest camps for salt traders along the routes through Ankole and Kigezi was abandoned for lack of demand.[52]

The salt traders may have been responsible for spreading relapsing fever along the hundred-mile route between Katwe and Kigezi during the 1920s, but there is reason to suspect that external factors triggered the process. Indeed, the Kigezi epidemic of 1923–24 was directly associated with the development of large-scale international migration of "temporary" laborers entering Uganda, principally from Belgian Ruanda-Urundi, but also from Tanganyika and the Congo. Most of this great flow of migrants, which swelled to include as many as 200,000 persons seasonally entering and leaving Uganda by the late 1940s, crossed into or out of the Protectorate via the famous Southwest route. This "route" was actually a combination of several streams of immigration and emigration across an essentially open frontier which extended eastward for 180 miles from the Ruanda and Congo borders with Kigezi to northwest Tanganyika and Lake Victoria. Controlled border crossings were established at Kakitumba Bridge and Murongo Ferry on the Ankole boundary, and at Kyaka Ferry on the Kagera River inside Tanganyika. Many hundreds must have also made their way into the Protectorate each year at unsupervised locations along the Kagera River. Upon entering Uganda the immigrants would spend a period of weeks or months making the journey on foot 75 to 200 miles into the fertile coffee, cotton, and sugar-growing areas of Buganda, especially Buddu and Kyagwe Counties, and of course Kampala. This migration was exceptional for its large scale and orientation to areas of small-scale cultivation. Its history and socioeconomic characteristics are examined in considerable depth in Richards' classic study.[53]

Temporary migration of thousands of Banyaruanda and others into Uganda annually along the Southwest route presented optimal conditions for the spread of a disease like relapsing fever. A

marked expansion in the size of the migration occurred during
1923–24. This change was linked to the introduction of compulsory cultivation of certain food and cash crops in Ruanda
by the Belgian administration, and was no doubt also a response to increasing demand for labor and a sharp rise in cotton prices in Buganda.[54] Concurrently, apprehension was growing
among medical authorities over the rapidly deteriorating health
status of the migrants. As early as 1926 the Governor of Uganda
considered barring recruitment of labor from the southwest until
health conditions in Kampala, which were causing "grave anx-
iety," improved. The Banyaruanda, in particular, were described
as "a miserably poor lot" and prone to malaria, relapsing fever,
and typhoid. Cases of relapsing fever in 1926 had exceeded those
of the previous year by more than 100 percent. Most of the victims contracted the disease in tick-infested resthouses and camps
along the main routes through Ankole and Masaka, which were
quickly becoming permanent foci of infection (see Figure 5).[55]
In Kampala, between 50 and 100 percent of the immigrant porters arriving there were said to have relapsing fever.[56] In Uganda,
the total number of reported cases shot up from 659 in 1925 to
2,494 in 1928, an increase of nearly 300 percent.[57]

Although systematic records of the number of migrants entering and departing Uganda by the Southwest route were not kept
before 1936, available estimates clearly point to a direct association between the initial surge of immigration from 1925 to 1929
and a dramatic outburst of relapsing fever. For example, from
1926 until the end of 1927 the number of immigrants using the
Southwest route increased by 290 percent and the number of
cases of relapsing fever by 203 percent. During 1928 the estimated number of migrants increased by 23 percent, while reports
of relapsing fever rose by 25 percent over the previous year to
reach the Uganda record total of 2,494 cases.[58]

Beginning with the mid-1920s we can document the first episode in a four-phase series of wave-like advances and retreats in
the prevalence of relapsing fever in Uganda (see Figure 4). A
similar pattern of less magnitude occurred in Kenya. Subsequent
peaks in the cyclical pattern in Uganda occurred in 1932–34

Figure 5. *Relapsing Fever in Uganda, 1931–55*

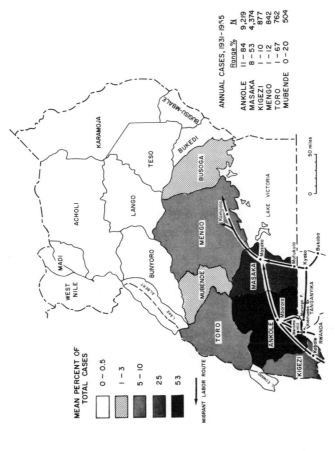

ANNUAL CASES, 1931–1955		
	Range %	N
ANKOLE	11 – 84	9,219
MASAKA	8 – 53	4,374
KIGEZI	1 – 10	877
MENGO	1 – 12	842
TORO	1 – 67	762
MUBENDE	0 – 20	504

MEAN PERCENT OF
TOTAL CASES

0 – 0.5
1 – 3
5 – 10
25
53

MIGRANT LABOR ROUTE

Sources: 1931–35: R. B. Heisch, *East African Medical Journal,* XXVII (January 1950); 1936–55: Uganda Protectorate, *Annual Report of the Medical Department;* and A. Richards (ed.), *Economic Development and Cultural Change* (Cambridge, 1954).

(average of 1,286 cases), 1944–46 (average of 1,295 cases), and 1950 (731 cases). After 1950 reports of clinical relapsing fever steadily tapered off so that by the mid-1950s the number of yearly cases had fallen well below 100. During the 1960s an average of under eleven cases were reported annually, and by the early 1970s Ugandan health authorities felt confident enough to state that the disease was "no longer a problem."[59] In retrospect, the three decades from 1925 to 1955 were the most significant in the recorded history of relapsing fever in Uganda. During this period there were an estimated 27,000 reported cases and apparently several hundred deaths among hospitalized victims.

Analysis of the disease statistics by districts for the period 1931–55 (selected because data are practically complete) reveals a high concentration of all Uganda cases (est. 17,500) in Ankole (53 percent) and the Western Region in general (63 percent). The next most important district was Masaka (25 percent) in the Kingdom of Buganda, which accounted for a third of all cases in the Protectorate during the 25-year period under review (see Figure 5). These aggregated distribution patterns do tend to mask a tendency for shifts to occur in the relative proportion of relapsing fever cases in Buganda and in the Western Region, predominantly in Ankole until 1953. Although the reliability of the data is problematical, the fact that an increase in the proportion of total cases concentrated in the Western Province is rather consistently matched by a proportional decrease of cases in Buganda, and vice versa, raises intriguing questions concerning the epidemiology and spatial behavior of this disease in Uganda (see Figure 6).

What was the nature of the relationship between *O. moubata*, relapsing fever, and the immigrants from Ruanda-Urundi? The answers are far from satisfactory since it is doubtful that the actual incidence of the disease will ever be known. There are indications that the Banyaruanda exhibited considerable immunity to the disease-bearing ticks present in their own country. In an attempt to maintain this immunity after arrival in Uganda, immigrants would carry their own ticks along with them in small boxes or in bedding rolls so that they might be bitten periodi-

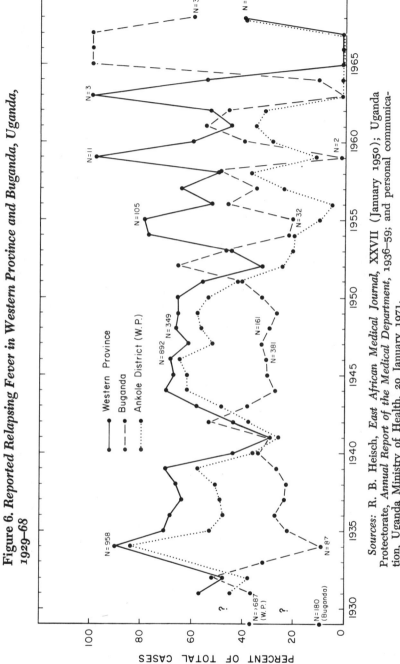

Figure 6. *Reported Relapsing Fever in Western Province and Buganda, Uganda,* 1929–68

Sources: R. B. Heisch, *East African Medical Journal,* XXVII (January 1950); Uganda Protectorate, *Annual Report of the Medical Department,* 1936–59; and personal communication, Uganda Ministry of Health, 20 January 1971.

cally.[60] This custom is also attributed to the Ngoni of southern Tanzania (who intentionally and ceremoniously placed ticks in a small hole dug in the floor of all new dwellings) and the Rundi.[61] However, the great majority of cases of relapsing fever recorded in Uganda occurred among the immigrant Banyaruanda.[62] As one might predict under conditions of sustained large-scale population mobility, an estimated 80 percent of the Ugandan cases occurred among males, in contrast to a slightly lower male preponderance elsewhere in East Africa. This pattern suggested "widespread concealed tick infestation" within Uganda and considerable immunity among the indigenous Ganda peoples who inhabited the immigrants' main target area. Banyaruanda, lacking cross-immunity, produced clinical symptoms of infection after being bitten by ticks harboring the local Uganda strain spirochete.[63] That the Ganda apparently did not often become infected with the Ruanda strain of spirochete suggests the social distance which separated them from their foreign visitors. This situation persisted even though many thousands of Banyaruanda took advantage of opportunities to settle permanently in Buganda, where they had easy access to *kibanja* tenancies under the *mailo* system. Although Banyaruanda were drawn to Uganda by the excellent possibilities for temporary wage labor, time after time the impetus for migration came from within rather than from outside Ruanda-Urundi. In 1948 Elspeth Huxley graphically described the background to this phenomenon.

The truth of the matter is that this comparatively small and once exceedingly fertile patch of Africa, Ruanda-Irundi—formerly part of the German East Africa but detached from it after the 1914–18 war and handed to Belgium under mandate—is grossly over-crowded. The population is reckoned to be nearly 3½ millions; that is, almost as many people are crowded into the 15,000 square miles of Ruanda as are spread out over the 94,000 square miles of Uganda. There are no industries to draw people off the mountainous land. The result has been as one might have expected.

Two years ago a drought came. Crops failed and, while thousands died, thousands more trekked to the green and fertile lands of Uganda. (People were shocked by the living skeletons they saw struggling along the roads, in some cases to die by the wayside.) The trek goes on. Last year, 140,000 people entered the Protectorate from Ruanda and only 4,000 went back.[64]

In addition to the periods of severe food shortages and the general scarcity of wage-earning opportunities, the flow of immigrants was quite sensitive to factors such as changes in the Congo franc-sterling exchange rate (increasing when the franc was depreciated).[65] Labor recruitment and health policies of the colonial administrations also exerted an influence on the volume of immigration, as for example in 1934 when strict quarantine measures were applied to both Tanganyika, because of sleeping sickness, and Ruanda, to control outbreaks of typhus, smallpox, and cerebrospinal meningitis.[66]

So-called "progressive" policies in Ruanda–Urundi also had a very noticeable impact on labor outflow. Thus, Belgian authorities explained the sharp 35 percent drop in immigration into Uganda between 1949 and 1950 in terms of the local commutation of labor dues, an increase in the price of African-grown coffee, and devaluation of the pound.[67] However, any cause-effect relationships between such specific events, immigration levels in general, and the pattern of relapsing fever in Uganda remain to be deciphered. Whether the apparent positive association between the disease and volume of immigration in the late 1920s was sustained over a longer period is not clear. Estimates of the actual numbers of immigrants are not available for 1933–35, but there does not appear to have been any significant change in the character of the migration. However, the years 1932–34 did constitute one of four peak periods in the known history of relapsing fever in Uganda. No less than 3,858 cases occurred during this time span, over 60 percent of them in Ankole. In 1935 there was an abrupt decline of more than 40 percent in total cases reported, yet the labor supply was "well-maintained throughout the year"[68] and the "increasing requirements of the sugar industry was reflected in a large increase in the number of applications to recruit, chiefly for Ruanda labour."[69] It is significant, however, that the Labour Inspector for Uganda, in his report for 1935, expressed grave concern over the shockingly poor standards of payment, housing, sanitation, water supply, rationing and feeding, and medical facilities which employers were providing for laborers at the cotton ginneries; in coffee, tea, and rubber plantations in Buganda; at the tin and wolfram mines of Ankole and Kigezi; and elsewhere.[70] Moreover, the inspector found existing facilities and the conditions along the Southwest labor route heavily traveled by Banyaruanda to be "thoroughly unsatisfactory."[71] Yet it was not until the late 1940s that British authorities, after several commissions of inquiry and years of procrastination, finally initiated a program to construct permanent rest camps and provide free rations for migrants using the Southwest route. For practical purposes this "progressive" development was too little and too late to effect improvements in migrants' health. By this time the introduction of bus service, the increasing use of private lorries, and the discovery of more effective chemical measures to control tick infestation had already begun to modify the pattern of relapsing fever in Uganda. Although there was a major outburst during the years 1944 through 1946, immigrants and Ugandan wage laborers (the Banyankore rather than Banyaruanda were said to "still form the largest proportion of all" African groups treated for relapsing fever at Mbarara) were increasingly able to by-pass the pedestrian rest camps infested with *O. moubata*.[72] The *Annual Report of the Labour Department for 1950* (p. 9) noted an "almost total swing over to bus travel," while the *Report for 1955* (p. 6) indicated that in a year characterized by a very large flow of immigrant labor it was "already an uncommon sight to see parties of migrants walking along the roads on their way to and from the centres of employment." Campaigns for systematic treatment of "relapsing fever houses"[73] and other African dwellings with benzene hexachloride (BHC) powder, changes in housing designs, and improved housekeeping methods such as adoption and maintenance of smoothly plastered walls and floors, had dramatic effects on the disease in Uganda and also in Kenya and Tanganyika.[74] The sharp but short-lived increase in relapsing fever in Uganda in 1959 (90 of the 105 cases occurred in Toro District, apparently at Katwe) is reported to be directly linked to a resurgence of tick activity following the application of BHC insecticide that had been incorrectly formulated (see Figure 5).[75]

Relapsing Fever in Kenya

From 1904 to 1910 Phillip Ross pioneered the investigation of tick-borne relapsing fever in Kenya Colony. Few cases were actually diagnosed apart from two infections from Fort Hall District and one from the Nairobi Bazaar.[76] Between 1911 and 1919 at least 109 cases were recorded. Although their precise distribution is unknown, these cases almost certainly occurred in one of the wetter highland areas which were soon to be recognized as the main centers of endemic relapsing fever in Kenya.

A majority of the 36 cases recorded in 1920 came from Ukambani. There is no account for 1921, but most of the 586 cases registered during 1922–27 occurred in Fort Hall District and Nairobi. Thereafter, the disease began to appear with consistency in the Jombeni Mountains above the 4,500 feet contour (focused among the Igoshi peoples),[77] and spread into Nyeri and Embu Districts around Mt. Kenya in the Central Province. In 1924 Shah discovered *O. moubata* in African roadside dwellings from Thika to Meru, and in 1927 Mackie observed that "relapsing fever is of common occurrence in this district (Meru) and many of the cases labeled *homa* (fever) by dressers at dispensaries are probably due to infection with spirilla."[78] Other endemic foci emerging at this time included the Taita Hills in southeast Kenya (above the 3,500 feet contour), Central and South Nyanza (Kisumu) and Kisii, and an area of low and sporadic incidence in the Digo District[79] south of Mombasa on the Kenya coast.

The trend of clinically diagnosed tick-borne relapsing fever in Kenya between 1925 and 1960 is shown in Figure 4. Cautious interpretation of these statistics as well as those for Uganda and Tanganyika is necessary, particularly for the earliest decades of colonial record-keeping. Before World War II there were very few hospitals. Absolute and relative distances were often so great that the populations living in very extensive areas were not effectively served and their disease profiles were unknown. Hence, it is not surprising that reports of disease activity in an area tend to follow the introduction of health facilities and the growth of awareness and interest and subjective definition of priorities by local medical authorities.[80] Thus in Taita District in Kenya there appears to be no mention of relapsing fever until 1927, the year the district hospital opened at Wesu.[81] Similarly, the concentration of cases in the Nairobi–Fort Hall area until 1927 reflects not only the intensity of African migration into this zone, but also undoubtedly the greater availability of health personnel, more disease surveillance, and comparatively well-developed medical facilities in the "settler core."

Investigations of *O. moubata* and relapsing fever during the late 1940s and early 1950s uncovered a classic example of the role of culture in cycles of disease transmission. The tick was virtually absent in the foothill zone of Mt. Kenya where people customarily slept on slatted wooden bedsteads raised on forked sticks driven into the cold damp floors of dwellings, and where goats and sheep were present to add their urine and trample the floors.[82] These factors created a very unsatisfactory microhabitat for ticks. The tick was abundant, however, in the neighboring and densely populated Jombeni Mountains of Meru District, which form a spur thirty miles long and twelve miles wide running from the northeast corner of Mt. Kenya. In this area of sedentary farmers, 40 percent of the houses had beds formed of a solid platform of mud with the head built against the wall and the foot secured by several superimposed logs only two feet from the perennial cooking fire in the center of the floor. Among the Igembi subgroup of the Bantu-speaking Meru peoples, this type of bed was found in 62 percent of 114 dwellings examined.[83] The cracks and crumbling parts of these beds near the fire harbored ticks in 25 percent of the houses. As Walton observes, the ticks' food supply "could scarcely have been nearer when the human occupants slept on these platforms."[84] In contrast, people such as the adjacent Tigania Meru used raised beds of wood slats in 92 percent of the houses examined, as did most peoples living around Mt. Kenya. There were far fewer ticks per house in these areas. And the incidence of infestation dropped below 10 percent when domestic animals were also present. Following these investigations the people of Meru district

were instructed to replace the mud beds with simple bedsteads and occasionally puddle the hut floors with water [to raise the relative humidity above the optimum for the ticks]. During the six years following the survey, hospital admissions diagnosed as relapsing fever in the two hospitals serving the area fell from a figure of approximately 300 per annum to less than five. A survey made in 1958 showed that the people had extensively followed the instructions and "*O. moubata*" had virtually disappeared.[85]

Certain Bantu peoples adopted rather shrewd techniques to shield themselves from contact with infected ticks. Such practices support Walton's belief that most East Africans recognize *O. moubata*, know about the disease it causes, and understand how to maintain immunity. Thus among the tick-free Kamba,

tribesmen living on the plains to the northwest in Kenya drove cattle from the north to trade to the Washambaa but on arriving at the foot of the Usambara mountains [northeast Tanzania] they sleep in the open. Sales transactions are carried out by resident Wakamba whose houses are tick infested.[86]

The decade of the 1950s brought dramatic results for campaigns against relapsing fever throughout Kenya. Although the number of relapsing fever cases in the district hospitals of Central Province showed a steady decline from 1952 onward, there was firm evidence in 1955 that the disease might soon be eradicated. Between 1952 and the end of 1955, the number of reported annual hospital cases fell from 115 to 9 in Nyeri, 50 to 11 in Meru, 67 to 3 in Embu, and 9 to nil in Fort Hall.[87] In addition to the successful preventive measures undertaken in Meru, the general decrease in the incidence of relapsing fever throughout the Central Province is seen by Teesdale as

a sequel to the measures undertaken by the Kenya Government to deal with the Mau Mau uprising and the declaration of the state of emergency in November 1952. The policy of bringing the peasant population into stockaded villages resulted in the evacuation of large numbers of huts infested with *Ornithodorus moubata* and caused a break in the transmission of the disease. This move alone would probably have proved of only temporary benefit had it not been for the institution of regular searches for ticks in the new villages. Some of these villages incorporated old tick-infested huts while in others ticks were introduced into new huts, presumably among clothing and bedding.[88]

Routine searches of dwellings by entomologists, immediate treatment of tick-infested dwellings with 0.5 percent Gammexane dusting powder, implementation of new housing and bed designs, and use of improved spirochetal drugs to treat the human reservoir of infection were key factors contributing to a reduction of 90 percent in the incidence of the disease in Central Province between 1952 and 1955.

Elsewhere in Kenya there were similar successes on a smaller scale brought about through government campaigns and by African vigilance and receptivity to control techniques. In the Taita Hills the number of reported cases decreased from 73 in 1953 to 3 in 1959. In western Kenya, where the incidence was normally moderate in comparison to Central Province, significant reductions in relapsing fever were recorded for Central Nyanza by 1952, North Nyanza by 1955, and South Nyanza by 1957.[89] In the Digo District of southeastern Kenya there were few cases of the disease after 1952. Conventional control measures, coupled with the fact that the ticks typically feed mostly on chickens in this coastal area of the country, reduced the disease to one of low incidence and sporadic occurrence.

Despite the few cases of relapsing fever diagnosed among inpatients of Kenyan hospitals since Uhuru in 1963 (an average of less than three per year), it would be unwise not to suspect a hidden reservoir of *B. duttoni* and ticks in old endemic areas of the country.[90] Since *O. moubata* can survive in dwellings for long periods without feeding there is always a possibility that the tick-man transmission cycle might be reestablished through the relaxation of hygienic conditions in the domestic environment, population movement associated with war or other disturbances (e.g., an epidemic of another disease), or climatic cycles.[91]

Louse-borne relapsing fever represents another though later health problem. The first recorded major epidemic of louse-borne relapsing fever struck Kenya at the end of World War II. Evidence suggests that this outbreak was indirectly linked in time and place with the great wartime epidemic which was centered in the Jabal as-Sauda area of the Fezzan in Libya at the end of 1942. From there it spread rapidly to the north and west, reaching Tunisia in October 1943; Algeria in November 1944; and Morocco in February 1945.[92] Spreading east, it reached Asyut in middle Egypt by October 1944, where 118,277 cases were recorded during 1945–46. Lebanon recorded 173 cases between 1942–46, Israel 600 cases in 1946, and Iraq 958 cases between 1945–47. Apart from Iran, which had 70,000 cases between 1945–47, other areas of the Middle East experienced less than the full brunt of the epidemic but nevertheless kept the diffusion process alive. Upon reaching Aden the disease spread to Seihut on the coast of southern Arabia, and from there to Mombasa, Kenya, in February 1945, apparently after the arrival there of a number of Arab dhows with infected passengers or crew aboard. The disease swept into the hinterland from Mombasa Island and by September–October of 1945 was particularly severe in the Giriama Reserve, where about 2,000 cases occurred with a mortality rate of 40 percent in untreated victims.[93] Control measures, including the use of DDT and restrictions on local travel, effectively controlled the disease in 1946.[94]

Writers commenting on the Kenyan louse-borne epidemic have apparently dismissed the possibility that the disease might have spread to the Coast Province via Moyale, a frontier administrative outpost on the northern border with Ethiopia. Yet in 1943 and 1944 there were 72 and 20 cases respectively of louse-borne relapsing fever recorded at Moyale which were believed "to come from Abyssinia."[95] In 1937 there had also been "an outbreak of what was assumed to be the same type of relapsing fever amongst Abyssinian refugees at Isiolo," which is located 250 miles to the southwest of Moyale and very near the main population center of Kenya.[96] Thus, while it is unlikely that the 1945–46 epidemic spread from Moyale rather than Mombasa, the fact that most medical references to the epidemic are noncommittal regarding its place of entry suggests the need for a more thorough analysis of archives at various localities within Kenya.[97]

Relapsing Fever in Tanganyika

As noted earlier, field studies by Dutton, Todd, and Koch during the period 1903–1905 clearly confirmed the presence and hazard of infected *O. moubata* at numerous locations along and off the old caravan routes from the coast to Tabora and Iringa via Kilosa. Annual medical reports for 1918–20 reveal relapsing fever to be widespread in the Mwanza and Musoma Districts of Lake Province, and record that a severe epidemic struck a detachment of the King's African Rifles headquartered in Mwanza.[98] This was apparently but one episode in a "major exacerbation" of relapsing fever in Tanganyika during World War I.[99] In contrast, the Medical Report for 1924 identifies southwestern Tanganyika as the most afflicted by "spirillum." Here, "drafts of troops and recruits were suspected of spreading the infection from Nyasaland northwards into Tanganyika; for *O. moubata* was extensively established along the main carrier routes, though the number infected was not large."[100]

By 1927, Tabora, located on the western plateau about 100 miles south of Lake Victoria, had achieved an unenviable distinction as the chief endemic center of relapsing fever in Tanganyika. Elsewhere the south-north routes in the eastern half of the territory was also discovered to be infected with *O. moubata*, although in 1929 there were only 354 reported cases of relapsing fever for the entire territory. Within three years this figure nearly doubled, and in 1933 the case load increased to more than 1,000 admissions. For the next 24 years the annual cases of relapsing fever would never drop below this mark; it reached a peak of nearly 6,000 cases in 1946 (see Figure 7).

During the interwar years and World War II, many up-country locations, including Mwanza and Kahama Districts in the Lake Province and Biharamulo in Western Province, as well as

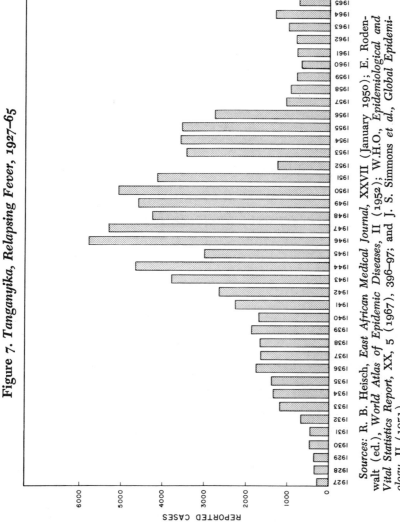

Figure 7. *Tanganyika, Relapsing Fever, 1927–65*

Sources: R. B. Heisch, *East African Medical Journal,* XXVII (January 1950); E. Rodenwalt (ed.), *World Atlas of Epidemic Diseases,* II (1952); W.H.O., *Epidemiological and Vital Statistics Report,* XX, 5 (1967), 396–97; and J. S. Simmons *et al., Global Epidemiology,* II (1951).

Kigoma, Shinyanga, and Maswa became heavily infested with
O. moubata and accounted for most of the known relapsing fever.
Coastal areas were to remain comparatively vector and disease
free.[101] A majority of the 3,000 cases in 1945 were in the Lake
Province, although by now the tick had been recognized in such
widely separate areas as Kileo near Moshi; and near Kongwa, the
location of the infamous agricultural development project known
as the Groundnut Scheme.[102] Overall, however, relapsing fever
remained most prevalent in the northwest of Tanganyika, despite
the far greater abundance of *O. moubata* in the arid, hot center
of the country. Tick infestation in the countryside south of
Dodoma, for example, was heavier than any other area investigated, there being large numbers collected in 95 percent of the
Wagogo houses.

During and after World War II, Tanganyika experienced a
dramatic surge of relapsing fever (see Figure 7), similar to the
pattern which occurred in Uganda and, to a lesser extent, in
Kenya during the same period. In attempting to identify some of
the causes of this phenomenon, one must rely less on medical
science and more on the concerns of social science. There is little doubt that the increased incidence of the disease was linked
to the marked growth of population movement in Tanganyika
occasioned by the war and the development of new wage-earning
opportunities. Military and economic factors were paramount.
Many army recruits who returned to their home areas during the
war soon found themselves being recruited once again, this time
for productive employment.

By 1945 an estimated 340,000 Africans were regular wage
earners in Tanganyika. A great many were migratory laborers
employed in large-scale agricultural enterprises such as the sisal
estates (attractive to veterans) in Tanga Province in northeast
Tanganyika, European mixed farms in the Northern Province,
and the Lupa goldfields near Mbeya in the southwest (some
20,000 men were working here in 1939).[103] Others were attracted
to the Williamson diamond mines at Shinyanga between Mwanza
and Tabora.[104] At the close of the war annual recruitment for the
sisal industry jumped from a little more than 2,000 men in 1945

to nearly 6,000 by 1952.[105] Whereas the extent of male absentee-ism in Tanganyika did not attain the high levels generally found in the Rhodesias and Nyasaland, a survey by the Labour Depart-ment in 1944 at Njombe in the southwest of the territory revealed that 46 percent of the men were absent from home.[106] Further evidence of the increasing mobility of Tanganyikans is found in the sharp rise in the number of third-class railway tickets pur-chased during the periods 1941–46 (from about 0.5 to 1.5 mil-lion) and 1947–51 (from about 1.3 to 2.5 million).[107] These and other developments created a very favorable milieu in which ticks and relapsing fever were easily spread from one area and population to another.[108] The process involved increased contact by nonimmune persons with old foci of infestation and endemic relapsing fever, as well as human dispersal of ticks and the in-troduction of exotic strains of the pathogen among populations lacking cross-immunity. Thus, during the period from 1946 through 1951, annual hospital admissions for relapsing fever averaged 4,842 cases. Curiously, in 1952 the incidence plum-meted to 1,231 cases, the lowest level since 1933, only to rise again to more than 3,400 cases in 1953 and over 3,500 cases re-spectively in 1954 and 1955.

Relapsing fever ravaged many of Tanganyika's town-dwelling populations, and it was there that the majority of the reported cases occurred before, during, and after World War II. In Morogoro, for example, the ticks and the disease were apparently carried to the sisal estates near the township by immigrant lab-orers traveling from Tabora to Dar-es-Salaam. Conditions in such towns were described as "hopeless" until Gammexane, a BHC insecticide first introduced in Tanganyika in 1948–49, could be applied on an extensive scale. However, Walton contends that because the disease was town-focused attention was diverted away from the rural origin of the ticks and infection and from the concealed reservoirs of ticks beyond human settlements.[109]

The distribution of BHC to many population centers was prob-ably the principal reason underlying the dramatic 70 percent decrease in relapsing fever recorded in 1952 (see Figure 7). By this time all infested towns were receiving routine applications of this insecticide, and its efficacy was soon proven despite ever-increasing African mobility.[110] Why, then, was there a sudden three-fold increase in hospital cases of relapsing fever during 1953 through 1955? The explanation appears to hinge, once again, more on the social behavior of man than on the tenacity of the vector. During this period there was a marked growth in the peasant-grown cotton industry in Tanganyika, particularly among the Sukuma people south of Lake Victoria. With their improved economic status, farmers greatly enhanced their mobility by acquiring bicycles, which they purchased in large numbers. Their widespread use in the Lake Province, then estimated to contain 280,000 tick-infested dwellings (90 percent in some areas), contributed substantially to the increases in relapsing fever recorded for 1953–55.[111] Meanwhile, the incidence of the disease in the Western Province tapered off steadily between 1949 and 1959. Most of the military recruits during the war were drawn from among the Nyamwezi people who inhabit this province. The continued decline of the disease here is thought to be linked to the sanitary instruction the Nyamwezi received during army training. "An examination of their homes," observes Walton, "would show that there had been a steady improvement in design, method of construction, and in details of housekeeping, with a slow improvement in standard of living."[112]

After 1956 there seemed to be a rather sharp decline in relapsing fever in Tanganyika. Fewer than 1,000 persons were hospitalized annually for a six-year period until 1964, when a relatively minor epidemic of unknown distribution occurred (see Figure 7). However, these figures can only hint at the true extent of the disease in Tanganyika. While there were 7,298 hospital cases and 175 deaths (a case fatality rate of 2.4 percent) from 1957–64, another 8,534 persons with relapsing fever were recorded as outpatients of hospitals or dispensaries during the period.[113] If only half of these outpatients were bona fide relapsing fever cases, the overall incidence for the period would increase by 58 percent. Likewise, if this figure is applied as a constant ("low-side error factor") for the entire colonial and postindependence periods, we are obliged to recognize what is potentially a vast hidden reservoir of infection in the human population of Tanganyika—and perhaps Uganda and Kenya.

We can merely speculate about the trend of relapsing fever since 1965. From this time onward no information is available in the customary source.[114] Circumstances suggest that Tanzania either stopped sending annual reports on the disease to the World Health Organization, or the W.H.O. did not publish the data it received. There is no reason to assume that the incidence has been reduced to a negligible level. It will be recalled that Walton estimated there were in excess of one million tick-infested houses in the country in 1964. Morover, there is evidence of a relapsing fever epidemic in neighboring Rwanda. Whereas only 323 cases were reported for Rwanda in 1963,[115] there were 1,951 cases in 1973 and 1,268 cases in the first five months of 1974.[116] This outbreak was probably fueled by Rwanda's close social and circulation links with Burundi, which was then suffering massive disruption of the countryside due to a genocidal civil war. The interaction of populations between Rwanda and Burundi, and between these two countries and western Tanzania (both Rwanda and Tanzania were sanctuaries for thousands of refugees from Burundi) surely must have dispersed relapsing fever across a wide area along their common borders.

Conclusion

Tick-borne relapsing fever has been a disease of numerous, predominantly agricultural populations in East Africa for centuries. The fact that the distributions of the vector and of the disease are often very different underscores the critical role which human factors—particularly mobility patterns, architectural design, construction materials, and domestic hygiene—play in the ecology of relapsing fever. Many of the intrusive peoples of pastoral tradition, such as the Luo and Nandi, are traditionally little affected by relapsing fever. This phenomenon is traced to their practice of plastering walls and floors in dwellings and high sanitary standards within the domestic environment. Foci of heavy tick infestation are historically associated with population groups whose house-types and housekeeping customs create an optimum vector habitat. In Tanzania the circular "m'songe" houses with thatched roofs which were widespread among Bantu-speaking people have been singled out, as have the rectangular flat-topped, earth-roofed "Tembe" houses widely found in the central and southern parts of the country. Ancient house types such as the temporary thatched beehive hut, and the pit dwellings once used in the Kenya highlands and still occupied in the Kondoa, Irangi, and Kilondo areas of northern Tanzania, have also been singled out for their attractiveness as tick habitats.[117]

During the nineteenth and twentieth centuries, population movement in East Africa occurred on a scale and with an intensity never before experienced in the region. The ivory and slave trade, inter-African and inter-European warfare, town development, resettlement programs, labor migration, road construction, the provision of government services, and introduction of the bicycle are among the more important developments which contributed directly or indirectly to the spread of disease. The historic regional pattern of relatively restricted and comparatively stable pockets of endemic relapsing fever was almost everywhere disrupted. Both tick and spirochetes were desegregated and dispersed into new areas. Often a population with immunity to its local strain of the disease would have little defense against the imported variety.

Following World War II the control of relapsing fever became a reality because of the development and widespread application of the relatively inexpensive insecticide, benzene hexachloride; progressive improvements in the design and construction of dwellings; and the adoption in certain areas of bedsteads and windows, and the elimination of domestic animals and chickens from houses. These fundamental practices made it possible, over a lifetime, for thousands of persons in Uganda, Kenya, and Tanzania to realize a slight improvement in their health standard. Continuation of these measures, coupled with regular surveillance by public health authorities, is essential if the low profile of the disease achieved in the 1950s is to be maintained.

Notes

1. John Melton Hunter, "On the Merits of Holism in Understanding Societal Health Needs," *The Centennial Review*, XVII (Winter 1973), 1–19.

2. W.H.O., *Weekly Epidemiological Record*, XLV, 24 (1970), 261.

3. W.H.O., *World Health Statistics*, XX–XXVII (1968–74). For a local study of descriptive and statistical interest see J. de Zuleuta, *et al.* "Finding of Tick-borne Relapsing Fever in Jordan by the Malaria Eradication Service," *Annals of Tropical Medicine and Parasitology*, LXV, 4 (1971), 491–95.

4. D. Livingstone, *Missionary Travels and Researches in South Africa* (London, 1857), pp. 382–83; 628–29.

5. E. Hindle, "The Relapsing Fever of Tropical Africa. A Review," *Parasitology*, IV (1911), 183–84.

6. A. R. Cook, "Relapsing Fever in Uganda," *Journal of Tropical Medicine*, VII (1904), 24–26. Cook first reportedly "identified" relapsing fever in Uganda in 1899. See W. D. Foster, *The Early History of Scientific Medicine in Uganda* (Nairobi, 1970), p. 84.

7. P. H. Ross and A. D. Milne, "Tick Fever," *British Medical Journal*, II (1904), 1453–54.

8. J. E. Dutton and J. L. Todd, "The Nature of Human Tick-Fever in the Eastern Part of the Congo Free State," *Liverpool School of Tropical Medicine, Memoir XVII* (1905).

9. The term *moubata* is a local Angolan name for the tick. Gerald A. Walton, "The *Ornithodorus Moubata* Superspecies Problem in Relation to Human Relapsing Fever Epidemiology," *Zoological Society of London, Symposium*, no. 6 (1962), 83–156; reference on p. 119. According to David Ordman, there is a great variety of African vernacular names for this tick, depending on locality. In Malawi, it is known as *kufu*. In Zambia, designations include *nkhufi, nkuswi, tambani,* and *inkoko;* in Tanzania, *itungu, ithou, vari,* and *ngage;* in Zaire, *bifundikala, bimpusi,* and *mouyata;* and in South West Africa, *oshilumati* and *enghopio. Kimputu* is found in East Africa together with the Swahili name *papasi.* In the northern Transvaal, the Bapedi call it *twakga;* in Bochem district it is *makadoela;* and in Mozambique it is *xirrota.* See "Relapsing Fever in Africa," *Central African Journal of Medicine*, III (September 1957), 352.

10. Oscar Felsenfeld, "Borreliae, Human Relapsing Fever, and Parasite-Vector-Host Relationships," *Bacteriological Review*, XXIX (March 1965), 46–74; reference on p. 54. As early as 1906, Koch warned Europeans never to use African huts and resthouses when traveling through infected country, and advised them to "camp at least 20–30 yards away from any such places." See Hindle (1911), p. 200.

11. Walton, "The *Ornithodorus Moubata* Superspecies Problem," p. 129.

12. C. L. Sezi, "Relapsing Fever at Masaka Hospital," *East African Medical Journal*, XLVII (March 1970), 176–78.

13. Gerald A. Walton, "The Ornithodorus 'Moubata' Group of Ticks in Africa. Control Problems and Implications," *Journal of Medical Entomology*, I (10 April 1964), 53–64; reference on p. 55.

14. *Ibid.*

15. Walton, "The *Ornithodorus Moubata* Superspecies Problem," p. 129.

16. Walton, "The Ornithodorus 'Moubata' Group," p. 53.

17. Ordman, "Relapsing Fever," pp. 348–52.

18. Infected *O. moubata* have been found in Kenya from sea level to 9,000 feet. R. B. Heisch, "Studies in East African Relapsing Fever," *East African Medical Journal*, XXVII (January 1950), 9.

19. Walton, "The *Ornithodorus Moubata* Superspecies Problem," p. 96.

20. Walton, "The Ornithodorus 'Moubata' Group," p. 54.

21. *Ibid.* Lack of cross-immunity to relapsing fever has been found between spirochetal strains only 48 kms. apart in Kenya. In contrast, Bray reported cross-immunity between malaria strains separated by 385 kms. in Liberia. Pp. 54–55.

22. See Paul W. English and Robert C. Mayfield, eds., *Man, Space, and Environment* (New York, 1972), pp. 116–18.

23. Alexander Alland, Jr., *Adaptation in Cultural Evolution: An Approach to Medical Anthropology* (New York, 1970), p. 49; C. Hughes and J. M. Hunter, "Disease and 'Development' in Africa," *Social Science and Medicine*, III (1970), 479.

24. Walton, "The *Ornithodorus Moubata* Superspecies Problem," p. 144.

25. *Ibid.*, pp. 144–45.

26. *Ibid.*

27. *Ibid.*

28. Dutton and Todd, "The Nature of Human Tick-Fever," p. 1.

29. See, e.g., John Ford, *The Role of the Trypanosomiases in African Ecology* (Oxford, 1971), p. 178; and John J. McKelvey, Jr., *Man Against Tsetse* (Ithaca, 1973), p. 42. Heisch, however, thought because Dutton was unconscious and blood smears were negative for spirochetes that cerebral malaria was indicated rather than relapsing fever. See Heisch, "Studies," p. 2.

30. Dutton and Todd, "The Nature of Human Tick-Fever," pp. 13–14. The map is found in this same article.

31. A point made by Walton, "The Ornithodorus 'Moubata' Group," p. 53, in connection with tick distribution maps compiled decades later.

32. R. Koch, 'Preliminary Statement on the Results of a Voyage of Investigation to East Africa," *Journal of Tropical Medicine*, IX (1 February 1906), 43–44.

33. See Charles M. Good, "Salt, Trade, and Disease: Aspects of Development in Africa's Northern Great Lakes Region," *International Journal of African Historical Studies*, V, 4 (1972), 568–77.

34. *Ibid.*

35. Hindle, "The Relapsing Fever," p. 188.

36. *Ibid.*, p. 189.

37. Foster, *The Early History of Scientific Medicine*, p. 83.

38. *Ibid.*, pp. 83–84.

39. Hindle, "The Relapsing Fever," p. 188.

40. Cook, "Relapsing Fever," p. 24.

41. Hindle, "The Relapsing Fever," p. 188.

42. R. U. Moffat, "Spirillum Fever in Uganda," *Lancet*, CLXII (1907), 208.

43. *Ibid.*

44. Uganda Protectorate, *Annual Report of the Medical Department, 1957.* (Entebbe, n.d.), p. 11; and *Annual Report of the Ministry of Health, 1960–61.*

45. Good, "Salt, Trade, and Disease," p. 552.

46. Foster, *The Early History of Scientific Medicine*, p. 83.

47. *Ibid.*, p. 85.

48. The Lamkin report (1908) concluded that the incidence of syphilis was

as high as 90 percent among the population of certain largely Bantu areas. H. B. Thomas and Robert Scott, *Uganda* (London, 1935), pp. 301–2.

49. *Kigezi District Annual Report for 1929*, Par. 13. Entebbe Secretariat Archives (E.S.A.). Also see map in Good, "Salt, Trade, and Disease," p. 573.

50. D.C., Kigezi to P.C., Western Province, Memo 220/42, 16 April 1929, file 169, Ankole Archives.

51. *Ibid.*

52. Good, "Salt, Trade, and Disease," p. 584.

53. Audrey Richards, ed., *Economic Development and Tribal Change* (Cambridge, U.K., 1954).

54. *Ibid.*, p. 30.

55. *Ibid.*, pp. 31–32.

56. *Ibid.*, p. 33.

57. Disease data based on Heisch, "Studies," p. 7; and Uganda Protectorate, *Annual Report of the Medical Department, 1935* (Entebbe, 1936), p. 18.

58. *Ibid.* for relapsing fever calculations, and Richards, *Economic Development*, pp. 29–41, for migration estimates.

59. Personal communication, D. F. Ibanda for Permanent Secretary/Chief M.O., Ministry of Health, 20 January 1971.

60. Walton, "The *Ornithodorus Moubata* Superspecies Problem," p. 145; and Uganda Protectorate, *Annual Report of the Medical Department for 1950*, p. 10.

61. Walton, "The Ornithodorus 'Moubata' Group," p. 62; and H. D. Leeson, "The Recorded Distribution of Ornithodorus Moubata (Murray) (Acarina)," *Bulletin of Entomological Research*, XLIII (1952), 409.

62. For example, see Uganda Protectorate, *Annual Report of the Medical Department, 1935*, p. 19; *1936*, p. 22; *1946*, p. 19; and *1949*, p. 17.

63. Walton, "The *Ornithodorus Moubata* Superspecies Problem," p. 145.

64. Elspeth Huxley, *The Sorcerer's Apprentice* (London, 1948), p. 203.

65. Richards, *Economic Development*, p. 49.

66. *Ibid.*, p. 39.

67. *Ibid.*, p. 48.

68. Uganda Protectorate, *Annual Report of the Department of Public Works, 1935*, p. 11.

69. Richards, *Economic Development*, pp. 39–40.

70. *Ibid.*, pp. 40–41.

71. *Ibid.*, p. 41, quoting Elliot Report, 1937, par. 3.

72. Uganda Protectorate, *Annual Report of the Medical Department, 1949*, p. 17.

73. J. K. T. Cherry, "The Prevention and Treatment of Tick-Borne Relapsing Fever with Special Reference to Aureomycin and Terramycin. Part I," *Transactions, Royal Society of Tropical Medicine and Hygiene*, XLIX (November 1955), 565.

74. Walton, "The Ornithodorus 'Moubata' Group," pp. 60–61; and Uganda Protectorate, *Annual Report of the Medical Department, 1952*, p. 14.

75. Walton, "The *Ornithodorus Moubata* Superspecies Problem," p. 148.

76. Heisch, "Studies in East African Relapsing Fever," p. 5.

77. G. Walton, "Relapsing Fever in the Meru District of Kenya," *East African Medical Journal*, XXVII (February 1950), 94.

78. Heisch, "Studies in East African Relapsing Fever," p. 5.

79. G. Walton, "Relapsing Fever in the Digo District of Kenya Colony," *East African Medical Journal*, XXXII (October 1955), 377–403.

80. E.g., clinical diagnoses of relapsing fever among outpatients were generally ignored in favor of recording only those (hospital) cases confirmed on the

basis of microscopical blood examinations. See C. Teesdale, "Tick-Borne Relapsing Fever: The Present Position in Kenya," *East African Medical Journal,* XLII (October 1965), 529. Between 1950 and 1961 there were 1,122 cases of relapsing fever recorded among outpatients of hospitals or dispensaries, and 1,492 "acceptable" cases. W.H.O., *Epidemiological and Vital Statistics Report,* XX, 5 (1967), 396–97.

81. C. Teesdale, "Tick-Borne Relapsing Fever: The Present Position in Kenya," *East African Medical Journal,* XLII (October 1965), 529.

82. Walton, "The *Ornithodorus Moubata* Superspecies Problem," p. 89.

83. Walton, "Relapsing Fever in the Meru District," p. 95.

84. Walton, "The *Ornithodorus Moubata* Superspecies Problem," p. 89.

85. *Ibid.*

86. *Ibid.,* p. 129.

87. Teesdale, "Tick-Borne Relapsing Fever," p. 530.

88. *Ibid.,* p. 531. For Kenya as a whole there is some disagreement in the case rate data used by Teesdale, Walton, and other sources such as W.H.O. for the post-1945 period. In all instances, however, a sharp decline in hospital admissions for relapsing fever is recorded by 1955. A graph produced by Walton ("The Ornithodorus 'Moubata' Group," p. 61) records 800 cases in 1945 (cf. 449 cases compiled from other sources) followed by a rapid fall to ± 345 cases in 1950 (in agreement with all other sources). In 1951 Walton records 400 cases (considerably higher than other sources) and labels this peak "Mau Mau," after which his graph dips steeply to 50 cases by 1955.

89. *Ibid.,* p. 533.

90. In 1960 and 1961 there were, respectively, also 64 and 97 cases of relapsing fever attributed to outpatients of hospitals or dispensaries. W.H.O., *Epidemiological and Vital Statistics Report,* XX, 5 (1967), 396–97.

91. During the colonial era incidence of relapsing fever was also shown to be "affected by the three to four year cycles of high and low seasonal rainfall." N. R. E. Fendall and J. G. Grounds, "The Incidence and Epidemiology of Disease in Kenya. Part III: Insect-borne Diseases," *Journal of Tropical Medicine and Hygiene,* LXVIII (June 1965), 39.

92. In the North African epidemic of 1942–47, which also spread to parts of French West Africa, Nigeria, British Cameroon, Sudan, and Eritrea, there were 290,000 confirmed cases and possibly as many as an additional 800,000 unconfirmed cases divided about equally between Algeria and Tunisia. For data see Anna C. Gelman, "The Ecology of the Relapsing Fevers," in Jacque May (ed.), *Studies in Disease Ecology* (New York, 1961), pp. 121–28; and E. Rodenwaldt (ed.), *World Atlas of Epidemic Diseases,* II (1952), Special Map 2.

93. Rodenwaldt, *World Atlas,* Special Map 3, shows the distribution and intensity with which different areas near Mombasa were infected in 1945. The most severely affected zone extended 5 to 10 kilometers outward from Mariakani, about 16 kilometers northwest of Mombasa.

94. Heisch, "Studies in East African Relapsing Fever," p. 6; and Fendall and Grounds, "The Incidence and Epidemiology of Disease in Kenya," p. 139.

95. Heisch, pp. 6–7. *O. moubata* was never found at Moyale.

96. *Ibid.,* p. 7.

97. Heisch, e.g., writes that "it is thought that the disease was introduced by dhow" (p. 6). Ordman, "Relapsing Fever in Africa," states that "it may have originated in the great 1942–1946 louse-borne epidemic of North Africa, but was *probably introduced* . . . when a number of Arab dhows arrived in Mombasa" (p. 350).

98. Heisch, p. 8.

99. Walton, "The Ornithodorus 'Moubata' Group," p. 54.

100. Heisch, p. 8.

101. Ordman, "Relapsing Fever in Africa," p. 353.

102. Heisch, p. 8.

103. Vincent Harlow and Alison Smith (eds.), *History of East Africa*, II (Oxford, 1965), 621 and 627.

104. *Ibid.*, p. 620.

105. Walton, "The *Ornithodorous Moubata* Superspecies Problem," pp. 145–46. Increased exposure to relapsing fever and other diseases was all too common in many of the target areas for migrants. Reports from some of the sisal estates and the Lupa goldfields "showed extremely low standards of housing, nutrition, and sanitation," Harlow and Smith, p. 628.

106. Harlow and Smith, *History of East Africa*, p. 628.

107. Walton, "The *Ornithodorous Moubata* Superspecies Problem," pp. 145–46.

108. Part of the explanation for the sharp rise in reported cases of relapsing fever during the war years may be related to increased attention to microscopical examination of blood slides among military personnel, in particular. In 1942 the number of microscopes in Tanganyika increased noticeably, and in late 1945 their use was apparently intensified again in response to the scare created by epidemic of louse-borne relapsing fever in nearby Kenya. Walton, "The *Ornithodorous Moubata* Superspecies Problem," pp. 145–46.

109. Walton, "The Ornithodorous 'Moubata' Group," p. 55; also see P. C. C. Garnham, "Susceptibility of *Ornithodorous* to Fire," *Kenya Medical Journal*, III (1926), 265.

110. Walton, "The *Ornithodorous Moubata* Superspecies Problem," p. 146.

111. *Ibid.*

112. *Ibid.* and p. 147.

113. W.H.O., *Epidemiological and Vital Statistics Report*, XX, 5 (1967), 396–97.

114. W.H.O., *World Health Statistics Report*.

115. W.H.O., *World Health Statistics Report*, XX, 5 (1967), 397.

116. *World Health Statistics Report*, XXVII, 3/4 (1974), 118.

117. Walton, "The Ornithodorous 'Moubata' Group," p. 60.

4

River Blindness in Northern Ghana, 1900–50

K. David Patterson

River blindness or onchocerciasis is one of the major health problems of northern Ghana and several other regions of Africa. The disease is caused by a parasitic filarial worm, *Onchocerca volvulus*, transmitted to humans by a black fly, *Simulium damnosum*, and infection may lead to progressive loss of sight and eventual blindness. In the 1950s surveys showed that approximately 30,000 people in northern Ghana, about 3 percent of the total population, were blind. Although trachoma, smallpox, measles, accidents, and other factors had accounted for some blindness, onchocerciasis caused the majority of the cases.[1] The World Health Organization has recently estimated that one million of the ten million inhabitants of the 700,000 square kilometer Volta Basin region are infected with *O. volvulus*. About 70,000 people are "economically blind" and "many more suffer serious visual impairment."[2] Important foci of onchocerciasis exist elsewhere in West Africa and in Central and East Africa, including extensive regions of Zaire and southern Sudan.[3] The disease, an unintended by-product of the Atlantic slave trade, is also found in Guatemala, southern Mexico, and Venezuela.[4]

River blindness, as the popular term implies, is not randomly distributed. It primarily affects populations living near swiftly moving streams, the preferred breeding sites of the insect vector. Villages near such watercourses may have adult blindness rates of as high as 30 percent.[5] A high incidence of infection and blindness, together with the sheer annoyance caused by biting swarms of the appropriately named *S. damnosum*, frequently leads to the gradual abandonment of river valleys and the retreat of the population for several miles, beyond the usual flight range of the fly.

This phenomenon has greatly influenced the population distribution of the northern districts of the Gold Coast. Population densities in the valleys of the Sissili, Kulpawn, Kanyanbiya, Morago, Red Volta, and White Volta rivers are very low and have been declining for the last few decades.[6] Population maps show strips of empty land along the rivers and "islands" of dense settlement away from the valleys.[7] People abandon fertile, well-watered farmland and retreat to higher ground. Crowding in these disease-free zones often becomes so great that even highly intensive agriculture cannot produce enough food to feed the people adequately. Pressure on the land frequently leads to insufficient fallow periods and serious soil erosion, causing further nutritional problems. Erosion may expose more rocks in stream beds or seasonal gulleys, thus providing new breeding sites for the vector. If a village does not move from an infected area, blindness progressively reduces the agricultural labor force and the active population may become too small to work the farms and keep back the encroaching bush. Lack of food weakens the people and the village gradually dwindles away.[8] Thus, onchocerciasis often causes profound and permanent changes in human ecology.[9]

Despite the important role onchocerciasis has played in the northern Gold Coast and other areas in West Africa, colonial medical services were remarkably slow to recognize the disease and its consequences. Indeed, as will be discussed below, the problem was not discovered in the Gold Coast until well into the 1940s. A World Health Organization Conference in 1954 revealed the seriousness of the situation in much of Africa and, recently, international campaigns have been launched to control onchocerciasis, especially in the Volta Basin.[10]

The larvae of *Simulium damnosum*[11] can develop only in water with a high concentration of dissolved oxygen. Thus, eggs are laid on stones or other attachment sites in rapidly flowing streams or in places where placid water courses are disrupted by rocks or other obstructions. Dam spillways and bridge pilings are often breeding places.[12] Adult flies feed on blood obtained by biting people, animals, or birds. Although the flies normally forage within a few kilometers of their breeding sites, *S. damnosum* has been known to fly 40 kilometers to feed, and females can travel as far as 85 kilometers to establish new colonies.[13] The flies disappear in the dry season, when most of the streams cease to flow. Adult flies may estivate, but dry season survival remains one of the mysteries of *Simulium* biology.[14]

As stated earlier, onchocerciasis is caused by a roundworm of the filaria group, *Onchocerca volvulus. Simulium* flies, the intermediate hosts, ingest microfilariae when they bite an infected person. Developmental changes in the fly produce a larval form which is transmitted to man, the only final host, when the insect feeds again. The developing worms migrate for a while in the subcutaneous tissues, but as adults they settle down in dense masses under the skin. The victim's body produces fibrous tissue which encapsulates the worm mass, forming an externally visible nodule from a few millimeters to several centimeters in diameter within a year after infection. Adult worms mate inside the nodules, producing microfilariae which escape and wander in the skin where they may be ingested by a biting fly. Infected persons can usually be identified by the presence of nodules; positive diagnosis is by microscopic observation of microfilariae in skin snips.[15]

Onochocerciasis is associated with a variety of pathological conditions. The microfilariae may cause severe forms of dermatitis,[16] including "craw-craw," an intensely itchy condition which is said to have driven some victims to suicide.[17] Infection of the lymph nodes is common, and some investigators have linked it to elephantiasis of the genitalia. It is possible that the disease causes other systemic damage, as microfilariae have been reported in a number of organs.[18] The most important pathological complications are, however, lesions in any of several ocular tissues, probably caused by the host's reaction to dead microfilariae. Ocular involvement does not occur in all cases, and damage depends on the duration and intensity of infection. Loss of sight is gradual; total blindness develops only after several years of progressive deterioration.[19] Onchocerciasis is a chronic, not a fatal disease, though many of its victims become totally disabled and have to be supported by their communities for years.

Recent campaigns against onchocerciasis have involved mass treatment of victims and attacks on the vector. Treatment is by surgical removal of the nodules and/or antihelminthic drugs. Nodulectomy is sometimes helpful, but only the encapsulated adult worms can be removed. Drugs such as suramin and diethylcarbamizine are usually effective, but they often have unpleasant and dangerous side effects and the patient may have severe reactions to the dead worms.[20] Therapy will aid individual sufferers, but the only hope for controlling the disease is to eradicate the vector. Intensive efforts are being made to eliminate *S. damnosum* by treating breeding areas with DDT and other larvicides.[21]

Skin lesions caused by onchocerciasis were first discovered in 1875 by J. O'Neill, who observed cutaneous damage and microfilariae in an African from the Gold Coast. The parasite was described in 1893 by R. Leuckart, who studied adult worms in nodules removed from Gold Coast Africans by a German missionary. J. F. Corson found *O. volvulus* in skin snips from prisoners in Secondi in 1922.[22] During World War I the Guatemalan investigator Rodolfo Robles demonstrated a relationship between onchocerciasis and ocular lesions. Robles suspected that *Simulium* species acted as vectors, and in 1926 his suspicion was proven by D. B. Blacklock, who showed that *S. damnosum* was an intermediate host in Sierra Leone. In 1932 J. Hissette, a Belgian working in the Congo, was the first to link onchocerciasis with blindness in Africa. A year later ocular onchocerciasis was identified in the Sudan.[23] G. F. Saunders investigated eye troubles in the northern Gold Coast in 1929 and 1932, but he concluded that nutritional deficiencies, not onchocerciasis, were responsible.[24] In Nigeria onchocerciasis was suspected as a cause of blindness as early as 1937, but nothing was published and no investigation was made.[25] Hyperendemic onchocerciasis was recognized as an important cause of skin and eye disease in the Tenkodogo region of Upper Volta in 1938,[26] but this research was not known to doctors in the neighboring Gold Coast.

Despite some progress, the extent and importance of onchocerciasis in Africa was almost unknown before World War II. In
the Gold Coast, where the parasite was first described, physicians
did not recognize until 1944 that the disease could cause blindness, and its impact on the population was not even suspected
until the late 1940s. Onchocerciasis did not appear on the Medical Department's list of reported diseases until 1953.[27]

The geographical focus of this chapter is the area of the Gold
Coast hardest hit by river blindness, the Northern Territories'
districts of Wa, Lawra (Lorha), Tumu, Navrongo (Navarro),
Zuarungu, and Bawku (Kusasi), which now constitute the Upper
Region of Ghana. Early instances of mass blindness and river
valley abandonment noted by medical officers and administrators
will be examined to show the distribution of onchocerciasis and
the beginnings of a dim recognition by officials before 1948 that
a serious problem existed. The discovery of river blindness in the
post-1948 period will be described and the disease will be discussed in the general context of colonial medicine in the Gold
Coast.

Scattered references in administrative documents show that
onchocerciasis was a serious problem throughout the colonial
period. Political officers occasionally noted extensive blindness
in particular areas or commented on dwindling or abandoned
villages in river valleys. At least a few medical officers became
aware of mass blindness in northern districts, but little research
was conducted until 1944. It will be assumed in the following
discussions of blindness and retreat from river valleys that onchocerciasis was endemic throughout the period in those areas where
it was later found.

The prevalence of "craw-craw," a dermatological symptom of
O. volvulus infection, was noted in Northern Territories as early
as 1907.[28] In 1912 the District Commissioner (D.C.) of Navrongo
reported extensive blindness. A medical officer, Dr. C. L. Ievers
investigated this in the Tumu villages of Pina and Tumdi,[29] but
his report, if one was made, has disappeared.[30] Two years later,
D.C. Poole observed that blindness was common in Tumu Dis-

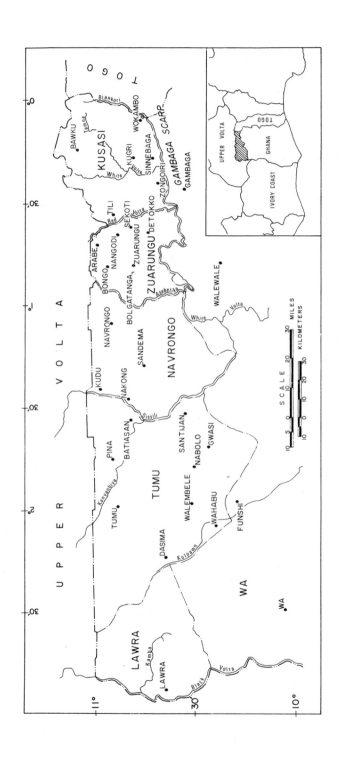

trict. He believed that flies spread eye diseases, yaws, and other afflictions.[31] The head of the medical services for the Northern Territories did not report blindness during his extensive tour of Wa, Lawra, and Tumu Districts in 1918,[32] but administrators in Tumu recognized that there was a serious problem. Michael Dasent noted in his 1918 report to the Chief Commissioner of the Northern Territories that "blindness is extraordinarily prevalent among the people of this district." He blamed this on the "dirt and swarms of flies which are found in every village."[33]

Blindness was reported in specific communities in Tumu District. In Dasima, an extremely dirty village near the Kulpawn, "it was very difficult to discover anyone who was not suffering from opthalmia, or terrible sores and ulcers, or other infirmity (*sic*)."[34] In Batiasan, another village, an "extraordinary" number of people were blind. The chief was sightless and his son was losing his vision. The D.C. speculated that this was caused by "the unsanitary conditions in which they live, especially the kraals of cattle in their compounds."[35] At Sapari and Gwossi, "every other person nearly, appears to be blind."[36] In the small village of Kachungmanjang in 1921, the D.C. reported that "the majority of the existing population is blind, owing to some contagious eye disease."[37]

Scattered through the Tumu Diary and Record Book are references to blind chiefs and headmen, for example, at Banan, Sinboro, Nmanjang, Kassano, Nabolo, Krubele, and Mapulima.[38] Many of these men were elderly and certainly some might have been blinded by trachoma or some other disease. However, almost all of the places with blind chiefs or where extensive blindness was noted were located within easy flight range of the Kulpawn and Sissili rivers and their tributaries—streams where *S. damnosum* breeds in abundance.

The census of 1921, the first serious attempt to determine the population of the Northern Territories, revealed high blindness rates in some northern districts.[39] The census taker in Tumu commented on the large number of blind people he encountered.[40] Among the 30,999 "Issalla Grunshi," most of whom lived in the Tumu portion of the newly amalgamated Lawra-Tumu

District, the census counted 1,164 blind people. This figure, believed to be an underestimate, indicated a blindness rate of over 3 percent. Venereal disease was suggested as a possible cause.[41] The census report for Wa made no mention of blindness,[42] but blindness was "far from rare" in the Northern Mamprussi District (Navrongo, Zuarungu, and Bawku).[43] Yet beyond this observation and occasionally noting a blind headman or chief, surviving records of the 1920s give few hints of the extent to which onchocerciasis was prevalent in Northern Mamprussi or in Lawra, Tumu and Wa Districts.[44] Perhaps this omission indicates less energetic or observant officials; or, quite possibly, onchocerciasis may not yet have been as serious as it was in Tumu where even there we find few post-1921 references because the district was attached to Lawra and was rarely visited by administrators. In all of these places, district record books were perfunctorily kept in the '20s and '30s. With one major exception, increasingly desk-bound district officials did not report extensive blindness or river valley abandonment in the decade after 1921. The exception was in Wa District, where a D.C.'s request helped to trigger an investigation of mass blindness.

The possible relationship between *O. volvulus* infection and eye disease was explored by Dr. G. F. Saunders, M.O. in charge of an experimental mobile health unit in the northwest. As was described above, *O. volvulus* was well known in the Gold Coast by the 1920s and by the late '20s, colonial physicians were aware that eye diseases were quite common in the Northern Territories. Dry season heat and dirt were thought to cause severe conjunctivitis with "corneal ulcerations leading to opacities and often to blindness."[45] In 1929 Saunders reported on unusual cases of blindness in Lawra and Tumu.[46] Three years later, at the request of the D.C. of Wa, Saunders investigated blindness in the Funsi area, and he observed that the condition was most prevalent where granite was common. Some Africans had thought certain rocks caused the disease. Saunders speculated that hard granite dust might cause eye irritations, but, not knowing that *S. damnosum* was the vector and that granite zones were associated with favorable breeding sites for the fly, he dismissed this theory.

Other local people "believed that blindness is caused by small nodules on the scalp."[47] Excised nodules were sent to Accra, where laboratory analysis showed that they were caused by *O. volvulus.* Saunders was aware that scalp nodules had been linked to blindness in Guatemala, but he found no correlation between either nodules or onchocercal skin lesions and eye damage in a sample of 75 from the village of Kulbaga. Instead, Saunders speculated that the blindness he observed might, like "night blindness," be caused by a vitamin deficiency. He suggested that people in the Funsi area be encouraged to raise and consume spinach.[48]

Although Saunders published in a major journal, his work was almost forgotten for more than a decade. Years later he concluded that onchocerciasis was a serious cause of blindness, but did not publish his conclusion.[49] He became involved in campaigns against trypanosomiasis after 1932 and did not follow up his early observations.[50]

The census of 1931 revealed a large number of blind people in the northern districts of the Gold Coast (See Table 1). Medical officers implicated dirt and irritations and some Africans blamed "certain grass seeds," but there was "no satisfactory explanation."[51]

Mass blindness was reported several times during the 1930s, but it was not linked to onchocerciasis. Dr. Stanley Batchelor, the M.O. for Lawra-Tumu, became interested in eye disease in 1934. On June 1 he was preparing to go to Tumu to investigate "the cause of the large percentage of blindness over on that

Table 1. *1931*

District	Population	Number blind	Blind/1000
Kusasi	110,614	903	8.1
Lawra-Tumu	93,125	771	8.2
Mamprusi	46,523	253	5.4
Navrongo	120,870	681	5.6
Wa	72,323	685	9.4
Zuarungu	133,981	322	2.4

Source: A. W. Cardinall, *The Gold Coast, 1931* (Accra, 1932), p. 226.

side."[52] Although delayed until early August by an attack of dysentery, Dr. Batchelor saw many patients in Tumu, including "a number of the 'eye' cases he wished to investigate, but unfortunately [he could] do nothing for them."[53] On August 16 the D.C. reported that Batchelor was back in Lawra but anxious to spend six months in Tumu during the dry season "and really investigate the cause of the great prevalence of blindness. At present he can only suggest that it is due to a dietetic deficiency of some kind."[54] Unfortunately, Batchelor was never able to continue his work in Tumu. In 1935–36 he was a popular M.O. at Navrongo, where he treated many eye cases, but he was subsequently transferred to Accra and never published his observations.[55]

Mass blindness was also reported in the 1930s in Bawku (Kusasi) District in the extreme northeastern corner of the Gold Coast. Although the Medical Department had almost ignored the district before 1932, health officials recognized eye diseases as a serious problem.[56] The D.C. for Bawku during most of the 1930s was J. K. G. Syme, an energetic, well-informed official with an interest in health conditions. Syme first became aware of extensive blindness in June and July 1936 when he toured the district to register taxable males. At Wokambo, a center in mandated Togo, he found that 97 out of 3,422 adult males (2.8 percent) were blind. Syme noted that:

In one small village of 9 compounds down by the river Morago, named Punkparyini, there are no less than four blind men and several blind children. In another section there are two compounds close together which between them contain five blind men and several blind children.[57]

The southern part of the district, toward the Morago River and the Gambaga Scarp, seemed to be hardest hit; in one section Syme found 9 men out of 232 blind.[58] At Sinnebaga his inquiries suggested a correlation between smallpox and blindness,[59] but the district M.O. blamed "conjunctivitis, probably fly-bourne."[60]

Syme returned to Wokambo in June 1938 and was alarmed at what he learned, especially in the sections closest to the bush along the Morago. His comments are worth recording in full.

Blindness seems to be increasing, especially in the three sections of
Bokko, Bulplise, and Sanwosi. In Sanwosi over 5% of the taxable
males are blind. It occurs mostly among the B'Moba part of the population and they are the people who penetrate furthest into the uninhabited country to make their bush farms. Ruins of former compounds
can be seen in some parts of the country but the Chief tells me that
nowadays one could not survive three years there without going blind.
It may be some fly-bourne disease, for flies are apparently very numerous as one gets nearer the Scarp, though we were not troubled by
them much on Sunday during our visit to the Dungu Turtle Pond.[61]

Furthermore, he observed that:

. . . blindness was again very prevalent amongst the B'Moba sections
and Gwoteri had over 5%. Blindness is far more widespread here
than tryps and I think it should be investigated. I mean to consult the
M.O. on my return to Bawku. In the meantime I have asked the Chief
to endeavor to have new cases of blindness brought in to Garu in the
early stages in the future. The section of Punkparyini, where both
blindness and tryps are common, now consists of five compounds only.
There were eight last year and more in previous years. I have instructed that no more compounds are to be built there until further
notice and no strangers are to go and live with the inhabitants already
there. This year several went and lodged there for fishing and have
remained on.[62]

Syme's report caught the eye of the Chief Commissioner of the
Northern Territories, who was anxious to learn the M.O.'s views
and wondered if dietary deficiency might be the cause. Syme
promised to collect patients for examination.[63] The M.O. began
work at Wokambo in January 1939, but he was interrupted almost immediately by an outbreak of cerebrospinal meningitis.
He thought that vitamin deficiency might be causing blindness.[64]

Thus, by 1939 officials realized that blindness was a significant
health problem in the northern districts of the Gold Coast, especially in Tumu and Bawku. Onchocerciasis was known, but its
relationship to eye disease was not recognized. Three doctors
worked on blindness in the '30s, but their results implicated
flies, dirt, and vitamin deficiencies, not onchocerciasis. Except for
Syme in Bawku, officials had not yet associated extensive blindness with river valleys. Meanwhile, across the border in modern
Upper Volta, a French investigator linked onchocerciasis with

blindness and river valley abandonment in 1938, but the out-break of World War II precluded possible intercolonial medical collaboration.[65] The British discovery of the importance of onchocerciasis was an entirely independent one.

River valleys in the northern Gold Coast have long been de-void of human settlement. Early maps show uninhabited belts along the streams of the Volta system,[66] and district record books, which often specify that a village is some distance from a stream, almost never mention a village actually on a river.[67] This was a puzzling phenomenon in a land marked by a long dry season and by occasional failure of the rains.

Prior to the discovery of onchocerciasis in the late '40s, colonial officials advanced several theories to explain the distribution of population. Early observers often blamed raids by Samori and Babatu.[68] However, there is no reason to suspect that raiders singled out river valleys for special attention, nor does it seem likely that these attacks, which ended in the 1890s, can explain population declines 30 or 40 years later.[69] Smallpox and cere-brospinal meningitis, two other explanations, did not selectively attack people living near rivers. Land exhaustion was another theory, but many abandoned areas were still arable.[70] Any or all of these problems could be locally important and might reduce a village below the strength necessary to be self-sustaining agri-culturally, but they cannot explain the overall situation.

Trypanosomiasis, like onchocerciasis, is transmitted by a vector which breeds near streams. In the 1930s sleeping sickness was considered an important cause of depopulation, and it undoubt-edly was a factor in some areas. The disease has been especially serious in the northwestern corner of the country.[71] A major epi-demic which swept most of Lawra and Tumu around 1886 de-stroyed many villages, particularly along the Kamba River.[72] In the 1930s the banks of the Kamba were uninhabited but dotted with the ruins of old compounds. K. R. S. Morris directed an ex-tensive campaign to clear tsetse-infested bush and to treat victims.[73] Sleeping sickness was indeed a serious problem in the Kamba valley, but onchocerciasis was also important. When the antitrypanosomiasis campaign was concluded in 1949, the gov-

ernment found people from overcrowded areas reluctant to colonize the Kamba region, despite "considerable inducements."
"On many occasions," reported the D.C., "I have been informed
by them that one of their fears is blindness. They state that people who have lived in this area have been bitten by little black
flies and gone blind; presumably they refer to onchocerciasis."[74]
Similarly, both onchocerciasis and trypanosomiasis were highly
endemic in the upper Kulpawn-Yelibifuo area. Antisleeping
sickness work was abandoned there when it became clear that
recolonization would be impossible unless river blindness could
also be controlled.[75]

Sleeping sickness was common in parts of Tumu, but even the
leaders of the antitrypanosomiasis campaign acknowledged that
the disease could not explain the alarming decline in population
and extensive abandonment of villages throughout the district.[76]
Political officers had almost ignored Tumu after its amalgamation
with Lawra in 1921, and the inhabitants of the district had received no medical attention. Depopulation was not discovered
until the early 1940s when a D.C. "deliberately sacrificed his
attention to Lawra District in order to get a closer acquaintance
with Tumu." The reasons for the problem were not clear, but
whatever the explanation, a dwindling population seemed unable
to feed itself.[77] Trypanosomiasis undoubtedly was a factor, but in
1949 B. Broughton Waddy showed that onchocerciasis was the
most important cause.[78]

The fact that local Africans were quite familiar with onchocerciasis and its consequences suggests that the disease had been
significant for many years. Former residents of the Kamba valley
were well acquainted with river blindness and clearly distinguished it from sleeping sickness. People in Funsi in the Kulpawn
valley associated head nodules with deteriorating vision;[79] they
sometimes had indigenous surgeons remove the nodules.[80] People
along the Red Volta, like Africans in Kenya and Zaire, associated
blindness and skin lesions with *Simulium* bites.[81] Fear of blindness prevented farming near rivers where the fly bred. Northerners avoided the rivers; practically all of the fishing was done by
migrants from the coast.[82] Hence, it is clear from early references

to blindness and from African knowledge of the disease that onchocerciasis had long been endemic in the areas where it was finally "discovered" in the late 1940s. And, although trypanoso-miasis and other factors could be locally important, it is evident that the major cause of river valley abandonment in the twenti-eth century has been onchocerciasis.

Early records provide some impressions of the extent and pace of population retreat from endemic foci. Oral data indicates that famine and drought propelled migrants to begin colonizing the banks of the Red Volta at Nangodi during the period 1890–95.[83] Prosperity prevailed in the well-watered and fertile land along the river until the years 1915–18, when, due to onchocerciasis, the population began a retreat which still continues.[84]

John M. Hunter has suggested that the settlement of river valleys in Nangodi and elsewhere in northern Ghana has fol-lowed a cyclical pattern of colonization of vacant land near streams, a gradual increase in onchocerciasis, and the eventual demise of the afflicted population or its withdrawal to higher ground out of the flight range of the vector. A growing popula-tion on a limited amount of land causes soil erosion and exhaus-tion in the watersheds; this in turn stimulates new attempts to settle the empty, inviting lands along the rivers. Memories of blindness in previous generations may well fade, and, indeed, the prolonged absence of people might have reduced or eliminated the *O. volvulus* population. Migrants might do well for many years, but the settlers would be vulnerable to a resurgence of the disease if infected flies or people came from other foci or if even a few of their own people retained living parasites. The attrac-tion of good farmland and the repulsion of disease may have caused a series of colonization/abandonment cycles over the cen-turies.[85] Perhaps data from future archeological research could be used to test this hypothesis.

While colonial records shed no light on the possible operation of such a cycle in the remote past, Hunter's proposed chronology for recent colonization and retreat does seem valid for Nangodi, Sekoti, and Detokko on the west side of the Red Volta. Oral evi-dence collected in 1935 indicated that Detokko was settled by people from Dusi, about five miles northwest, two generations before the arrival of the British in 1907. There were only three compounds in the area when the migrants came, perhaps around 1870.[86] Sekoti was settled in the 1880s, one generation before the British came. Here the newcomers found only empty bush to greet them.[87]

As early as 1907 a touring official found that the chief of Nangodi was old and blind; onchocerciasis may have already been a problem.[88] In 1908 the compounds of Sekoti extended to the river[89] and by 1917 land along the river in the Nangodi–Sekoti area was thickly settled. "All of this part of the country right down to the Volta is being built on and farmed now" reported S. D. Nash. "One can see the houses, etc., are of recent date."[90] Land in Detokko was also being rapidly occupied and compounds were scattered almost as far as the river.[91] The area just west of the confluence of the Red and White Voltas was attracting migrants during the same period. There were only a few scattered compounds in 1909, but four years later people from as far away as Bongo, Zuarungu Town, and Bolgatanga were moving in.[92] Immigration was still significant in 1917.[93]

It is difficult to date the beginning of the retreat from the Red Volta and the villages in the bend of the White Volta, because district diaries and record books became increasingly uninformative in the 1920s and the census of 1921 was not very detailed or accurate. In 1929 an official reported good hunting along the Red Volta at Nangodi; this observation suggests that significant retreat had already taken place.[94] Census figures for 1931 and 1948 indicate a progressive retreat from the rivers.[95] By the late 1940s the villages in the bend of the White Volta were dead or dying.[96] Nangodi, Sekoti, and the villages opposite them were all three or four miles back from the Red Volta; north of Nangodi the line of settlement had retreated even further.[97]

Surprisingly, despite the existence of a government resthouse and ferry at Nangodi and the activities of a private gold mine there in the 1930s, significant blindness was not reported anywhere along the Red Volta. The census of 1931 reported only 24 blind people at Nangodi out of a total population of 10,389.[98]

District commissioners and medical officers visited the area frequently, but they reported nothing unusual. By the 1940s at Nangodi people were trying to stay away from the river, but the village did have to provide ferrymen. These men were exposed to *Simulium* bites and usually contracted river blindness.[99] Although touring officials constantly used the Nangodi ferry, there was no reference to visually handicapped ferrymen until 1943 when, in the presence of the D.C. of Bawku, a blind collector dropped his tickets and coins and tripped over an eight gallon can.[100] The ferry had a reputation for inefficiency, perhaps because the operators were losing their eyesight.[101]

Similar evidence of settlement and retreat can be found in southern Bawku District, especially near the White Volta and its tributaries, the Tamne and the Morago. Much of this area, including the cantons of Wokambo, Sinnebaga, Kugri, and Zongoiri, was almost uninhabited bush at the beginning of the twentieth century. Some areas had once been populated, but Chokossi and Zabarima raiders had killed or displaced the people.[102]

Wokambo was almost empty until the 1920s, when Moba from French Togo began to settle in large numbers.[103] The population grew from 2,361 in 1921 to over 10,000 in 1931.[104] Some colonists pushed toward the Morago River and its tributary, the Biankuri. In 1929 a small Moba village was being built in the extreme southeast, a mile west of the Dungu Turtle Pond; the Sanvosi section on the Biankuri grew from 23 compounds in 1921 to 82 in 1933.[105]

The newcomers were suffering from onchocerciasis by the 1930s; the disease may have been already present among the small original population.[106] As was described above, J. K. G. Syme discovered extensive blindness in Wokambo and its western neighbor, Sinnebaga, in 1936. Two years later he found that blindness was increasing and was, as the people were well aware, most prevalent among those who lived closest to the rivers. Ruins of compounds showed that retreat had already begun in some places. The land around the Dungu Turtle Pond was now completely uninhabited and the Punkparyini section was being abandoned.[107] Other evidence is meager, but a 1928 map of Kusasi and a 1940 sketch map of Wokambo both show a large uninhabited area in the far southeast and ruins a mile north of the Turtle Pond.[108] Several sections where Syme reported extensive blindness suffered a substantial decline in population between 1931 and 1948.[109]

Scattered references suggest similar abandonment of river valleys elsewhere in Bawku. At Zongoiri, Syme observed in 1936 that "a good many people appear to have moved to other places."[110] Three small sections at Kugri were deserted between 1921 and 1929.[111] By 1945 old Kugri sections north of the Tamne were empty and areas of ruined compounds were evident there and in parts of Sinnebaga. The situation looked "very much like parts of Sekoti." The land did not seem exhausted; the D.C. could only speculate that there might be a political explanation, such as people fleeing an unpopular chief.[112] Four years later Dr. B. B. Waddy showed that the whole Kugri-Wokambo region was heavily infected with river blindness.[113]

Data on the northwestern districts are scanty. Near the Sissili River in northwest Navrongo, population decline, land abandonment, and crop failures were observed in Nakong and Kudu in the late 1930s. River blindness was widespread; the disastrous situation which Waddy later described in 1948 was already developing.[114]

Blindness was frequently described in early Tumu records, and the District Diary and Record Book repeatedly mention abandoned or dying villages in the Sissili and Kulpawn valleys. Mimojan, once a big town near the Sissili, was almost empty in 1917, although at Santejan soil exhaustion was forcing people to migrate to fertile lands near the Sissili.[115] Village abandonment was sometimes blamed on people moving to avoid road work, but the inhabitants of Wahabu, an important ferry crossing on the Kulpawn, left their homes because there was too much sickness and death.[116]

Retreat from the Kulpawn and Sissili valleys has been widespread since at least 1921.[117] Indeed, it seems probable that retreat began in the late nineteenth century. The first detailed map of the region (made in 1905) showed extensive uninhabited strips along both rivers.[118] An early British visitor to the mid-Kulpawn area in extreme southeastern Wa described a well-farmed region with many towns, but elsewhere in the Kulpawn valley and near the western tributaries of the Sissili, a contemporary observer described a fertile, well-watered, but sparsely populated countryside.[119] Except for Funsi and a few other towns, the land was empty or marked only with ruined villages.[120] Conditions in modern Tumu suggest that population retreat and land exhaustion have gone on longer there than in other districts.[121]

The first published suggestion that onchocerciasis caused extensive blindness was made in 1940 by Dr. F. M. Purcell, who was conducting a survey of rural nutrition in the northeast. At first Purcell thought that most blindness in the region was due to a deficiency of vitamin A, but further observations and a study of the writings of Hissette and other workers convinced him that *O. volvulus* infection was "the principal cause of blindness in the north." The disease seemed worst among those who fished in the Sissili River.[122] Nakong, on the east side of the Sissili, suffered badly; Purcell believed that onchocercal blindness was at least partially responsible for the chronic famine conditions which prevailed there.[123] He recommended studies of the vector and the distribution of the disease, evacuation of heavily infected areas, discouragement of fishing in the Sissili, and the establishment of traveling dispensaries to treat victims.[124]

Purcell's comments on onchocerciasis probably helped to pave the way for Dr. Harold Ridley's research which, in 1944, first showed the social and medical significance of the disease. Ridley, a government ophthalmologist stationed at the military hospital in Accra, was struck by the high incidence of eye disease among soldiers from the Northern Territories. He associated this with onchocerciasis and communicated with Dr. Saunders, who now believed that onchocerciasis was responsible for the blindness he had described in 1933. Armed with data from Saunders and supplied with patients by Dr. Waddy, M.O. of the 1st Battalion of the Gold Coast Regiment, Ridley realized that he had stumbled across a serious problem.[125] In July 1943 he applied for leave and funds to conduct research in the north.

Delayed by the press of wartime duties, Ridley did not reach the north until February 1944. He chose to work at Funsi, the site of Saunders's earlier work. He found onchocercal nodules in 131 of the 300 people surveyed. One hundred forty-one persons were given ocular examinations; 51 had damage caused by *O. volvulus* and 10 suffered from other eye diseases.[126] Ridley, the first eye specialist to work in the north, conclusively demonstrated the link between onchocerciasis and mass blindness.

Ridley's conclusions attracted governmental attention at the highest level. The Director of Medical Services realized that onchocerciasis had to be a target of postwar health campaigns. "There is no doubt that it [onchocerciasis] is fairly widespread and that a considerable amount of blindness results."[127] Governor Alan Burns agreed that the disease required attention, but he took no action against it in the immediate postwar period because of "the acute staff shortage."[128] River blindness was ignored until 1948, when the work of Dr. Waddy forced the Medical Department to take action.

Waddy had been M.O. for Lawra-Tumu in 1939 "without the faintest suspicion that hyperendemic, blinding oncho existed."[129] He first became interested in the disease in 1942, when he referred soldiers with eye problems to Ridley. Eager to investigate river blindness, Waddy volunteered to return to the north in 1945. However, he was the sole M.O. for a 14,000 square mile region in the north; in addition to routine duties, he had to contend with cerebrospinal meningitis and smallpox epidemics through 1946.[130] After a year of study in England for a diploma in public health, Waddy returned to the Gold Coast in 1948 as Medical Officer of Health for the Northern Territories.[131]

The census of 1948, like those of 1921 and 1931, revealed significant blindness in the northern districts. In Wa, census-taking in January showed that "in certain places as many as 30% of the population are blind."[132] The M.O. for Navrongo, M. H. Hughes, used newly gathered data to show a correlation between high blindness rates and stagnant or declining populations. Nakong, the area worst hit, had an officially reported blindness rate of

6.5 percent; its population dropped 15.6 percent between 1931 and 1948.[133]

Waddy's first investigation of river blindness was at Tili, on the east bank of the Red Volta, in May 1948. He found *Simulium* breeding, extensive *O. volvulus* infection, and 23 out of 210 infected people either blind or with very weak vision.[134] Aware of Hughes's data, Waddy then turned to Nakong, where he found a shocking situation. *Simulium* swarmed all over the area, skin snips showed that almost the entire population harbored the parasite, and of the 1,074 people counted in the census 90 could see nothing at a distance of 30 feet and many others were nearly sightless. Several sections near the Sissili were deserted; many of the former inhabitants had chosen to die rather than move. The survivors seemed lethargic and were unable to protect their fields from wild animals. "The economic and social plight of the inhabitants could hardly be worse," wrote Waddy. "They are gradually fading out in disease and semi-starvation. . . . Such is the state of manpower in Nakong that the blind are led out to hoe in the fields." Onchocerciasis was clearly the primary cause of blindness; the rarity of nightblindness and the relative abundance of green vegetables seemed to preclude a deficiency of vitamin A.[135]

Determined to rouse the political and medical establishments, Waddy painted a bleak picture of the impact of onchocerciasis on the north.

Nakong and the Sissili area in general has 'had it.' No regeneration is possible. The people probably won't emigrate and they may not last another ten years. Around the Red Volta and much of the Kulpawn River the people are gradually retreating rather than dying off.

Intensive farming caused soil erosion, which exposed rocks and provided more breeding places for the fly. Important foci of the disease also existed along the Black Volta.[136]

Waddy then turned his attention to Nangodi which, until the completion of a bridge in 1946, had been an important ferry point on the Red Volta.

The working life of a ferryman here (I am credibly informed) was about two years; he then returned home blind and with his skin on fire with craw craw. These men are sitting about in Nangodi and probably in Tili, a drain on the community (if the community chooses to feed them) and a burden to themselves. The appointment of ferryman was not pensionable. It is my intention to get the statistics of this industrial disease as soon as I can; I mention it now to draw attention to the fact that onchocerciasis is no joke to its victims.[137]

The strongly worded Nakong report supported a proposal for a major survey of northern river valleys which Waddy had submitted in May 1948.[138] This proposal received no encouragement from the head of the medical services in the Northern Territories; onchocerciasis was a "cold" disease, at least in comparison to smallpox and cerebrospinal meningitis.[139] Eventually, however, a scaled-down investigation was authorized and Waddy, aided by African assistants, surveyed several carefully selected locations in April and May 1949.

Waddy's final report, based on data gathered in 1948 and 1949, is a landmark in the medical history of Ghana. He reviewed the literature on onchocerciasis. Although admittedly not an entomologist, he plotted the distribution of the vector and described its habits and breeding behavior. He surveyed sample villages in the Black Volta, Kulpawn, Sissili, Asebelika, Red Volta, and White Volta valleys for infection and ocular problems, and he showed that the 1948 census underestimated blindness rates. Onchocerciasis was clearly identified as a major cause of blindness and retreat from river valleys.[140] Although the report was not published,[141] it was no longer possible to ignore river blindness. The disease had been discovered.

Events moved rapidly after 1949. French investigators were working on onchocerciasis in Upper Volta[142] and, belatedly, medical contacts developed across the colonial frontier.[143] Newly established medical field units toured the north, looking for and treating onchocerciasis and a host of other diseases.[144] Meanwhile Waddy, aware of his lack of special training in ophthalmology, helped convince the Medical Department to send the government opthalmologist at Accra, Dr. J. W. R. Sarkies, to study eye disease in the north.[145] Sarkies confirmed the importance of onchocercal blindness and found the situation "most depressing."[146] Major ophthalmological and entomological investigations were begun late in 1952, although under the sponsorship of a private organization, the British Empire Society for the Blind, rather than the Gold Coast government.[147] The struggle against river blindness, begun in the early '50s, shows no sign of reaching a conclusion.

Except for treating eye and skin symptoms of a few people, the colonial government did nothing to combat onchocerciasis before 1950. Indeed, it is possible that the British inadvertently created conditions favorable at least to local spread of the disease. The population of the districts which now comprise the Upper Region of Ghana roughly doubled between 1921 and 1948.[148] Colonial medical services almost certainly contributed something to this growth, which put greater pressure on arable land and perhaps forced people to colonize or remain in endemic areas.

Colonial improvement schemes also helped spread river blindness. Ferries were maintained at major river crossings and, as at Nangodi, the operators were exposed to the disease. Bridge pilings and abutments and dam spillways often provided breeding sites for *S. damnosum* and thus created new foci of onchocerciasis.[149] This was observed at a dam near Tumu town in the early 1950s.[150] There was little major construction in the north due to lack of interest and funds, but during the 1930s development-minded D.C.s prodded local native authorities to build small earth dams. In Bawku, J. K. G. Syme had dams built in a number of places, including two areas affected by river blindness, Sinnebaga and Zongoiri.[151]

How did onchocerciasis go undetected for so long? "It is fantastic," Waddy later wrote, "that blindness on the scale of up to ten percent of the population in some villages should go unnoticed, or if noticed, disregarded, until the 1940s, but that is the plain unvarnished truth."[152] One factor was the shortage of staff in the north. Prior to 1945 there were rarely more than two to four doctors in the northern tier of districts; these overworked men had to cover huge tracts of difficult country and had little time for research or reading. In the prewar period not one doctor volunteered for a second tour of duty in the north. Physicians sought to escape from remote bush stations with heavy case loads and few facilities to more comfortable postings in the towns of the south.[153] Many districts, including heavily afflicted Tumu, had no resident doctor for years at a time and were served only by an occasional itinerant M.O. or antitrypanosomiasis team. Indeed, much of the feeble medical effort in the north was directed against sleeping sickness, especially in the 1930s. Furthermore, perhaps because of fear, fatalism, or the long travel time from some river blindness foci to district stations, few African victims sought medical aid.[154]

Equally important, even when colonial physicians were aware of high blindness rates in certain villages, they did not detect a pattern; instead they saw only isolated phenomena, easily forgotten in a sea of epidemic and endemic diseases. Doctors were simply not looking for onchocerciasis. They were aware that the disease existed in the Gold Coast but, despite work in Central America and the Congo, did not associate what seemed to be a minor skin disease with progressive loss of sight. However, if men who began investigations in 1932, 1934, and 1939 had not been interrupted by sleeping sickness work, transfer to the south, and a cerebrospinal meningitis epidemic respectively, the role of onchocerciasis might have been discovered years before the studies of Ridley, Hughes, and Waddy. The lack of contact between colonial medical departments, especially during the Vichy period, meant that French work in Upper Volta was unknown in the adjacent Gold Coast for more than a decade.[155] When Waddy finally demonstrated that onchocerciasis caused massive blindness and extensive land abandonment, colleagues could only join him in wondering how things which suddenly seemed obvious had gone unrecognized for so long.

Compared to the Congo, Sudan, and Upper Volta, the Medical Department of the Gold Coast was late to identify river blindness, although not as late as Nigeria.[156] Erroneous preconceptions of the nature of onchocerciasis and poor scientific communications help to explain why river blindness was ignored for so long in the Gold Coast. More significantly, the disease flourished in a remote section of the colony which was weakly administered and poorly served by the medical establishment. An official admission that Frafra country in the northeast was "very little known . . . from the medical point of view until after the war" is true for the entire region.[157] The failure to recognize onchocerciasis was only one example of the hazy knowledge of health conditions in the far north.

Notes

Research for this chapter was supported by NIH Grant LM02517 from the National Library of Medicine.

1. F. C. Rodger, *Blindness in West Africa* (London, 1959), pp. 89–90, 93; B. B. Waddy, "Onchocerciasis and Blindness in the Northern Territories of the Gold Coast," unpublished report, 1949, p. 34. I am grateful to Dr. Waddy for a copy of this document.

2. World Health Organization, "Communicable Disease and Vector Control in 1973," *W.H.O. Chronicle*, XXVIII (1974), 322. The Volta Basin includes most of Ghana and Upper Volta and portions of Togo, Dahomey, Niger, Ivory Coast, and Mali.

3. W.H.O. Expert Committee on Onchocerciasis, Second Report (Geneva, 1966), map p. 7.

4. *Ibid.*, map p. 8; R. Hoeppli, *Parasitic Disease in Africa and the Western Hemisphere: Early Documentation and Transmission by the Slave Trade* (*Acta Tropica*, supplement 10, Basel, 1969), 139–42.

5. B. B. Waddy, "Prospects for the Control of Onchocerciasis in Africa with Special Reference to the Volta Basin," *Bulletin of the W.H.O.*, XL (1969), 843.

6. T. E. Hilton, "Frafra Resettlement and the Population Problem in Zuarungu," *Bulletin de l'Institut Fondamental d'Afrique Noire*, sér. B, XXII (1960), 430–31; Hilton, "The Settlement Pattern of the Tumu District of Northern Ghana," *Bull. I.F.A.N.*, sér. B, XXX (1968), 871–78; John M. Hunter, "River Blindness in Nangodi, Northern Ghana: A Hypothesis of Cyclical Advance and Retreat," *Geographical Review*, LVI (1966), 405–13; Alfred A. Buck, "River Blindness—Onchocerciasis—A Multidisciplinary Approach for Research and Control." *Transactions of the American Academy of Ophthalmology and Otolaryngology*, LXXIX (1975), 461–64.

7. Waddy, "Control of Onchocerciasis," p. 844; T. E. Hilton, *Ghana Population Atlas* (Edinburgh, 1960), pp. 6–10; Hunter, "Geographical Aspects of Onchocerciasis Control in Northern Ghana," unpublished report, World Health Organization (1972, 43p.), pp. 2, 3, 24, 25, 38, 40. I am grateful to Dr. Hunter for a copy of this report.

8. Hilton, *Population Atlas*, p. 26; Hilton, "Le Peuplement de Frafra, district du Nord-Ghana," *Bull. I.F.A.N.*, sér. B, XXVII (1956), 684–92; Hunter, "Nangodi," pp. 409–10; Hunter, "Population Pressure in a Part of the West African Savanna: A Study of Nangodi, Northeast Ghana," *Annals of the American As-*

sociation of Geographers, LVII (1967), 102–9; Waddy, "Control of Onchocerciasis," pp. 844–45.

9. Similar problems have been noted elsewhere in West Africa. See, for example, F. H. Budden, "The Epidemiology of Onchocerciasis in Northern Nigeria," *Transactions of the Royal Society of Tropical Medicine and Hygiene,* L (1956), 366–78; H. J. Knüttgen, "Remarks on the Epidemiology and Importance of Onchocerciasis in Upper Guinea," *Annales de la société belge de médecine tropicale,* LI (1971), 611–14; M. Lamontellerie, "Resultats d'enquêtes sur les filarioses dans l'ouest de la Haute-Volta (Cercle de Banfora)," *Annales de parasitologie humaine et comparée,* XLVII (1972), 783–838.

10. W.H.O., "Communicable Diseases and Vector Control in 1973," p. 314.

11. The black fly *S. damnosum* is a familiar pest in parts of the U.S and Canada. *S. naevi* is the vector in eastern Africa.

12. W.H.O. Expert Committee, Second Report, p. 10; G. Crisp, *Simulium and Onchocerciasis in the Northern Territories of the Gold Coast* (London, 1956), pp. 42, 49.

13. W.H.O. Expert Committee, Second Report, p. 11.

14. *Ibid.,* pp. 63–65; Crisp, *Simulium and Onchocerciasis,* pp. 11.

15. Edward K. Markell and Marietta Voge, *Medical Parasitology* (3rd ed., Philadelphia, 1971), pp. 255–60; Geoffrey Lapage, *Animals Parasitic in Man* (rev. ed., New York, 1963), pp. 101–3.

16. A. A. Buck, ed., *Onchocerciasis: Symptomatology, Pathology, Diagnosis* (Geneva, 1974), pp. 10–13.

17. Waddy, "Control of Onchocerciasis," p. 843.

18. Buck, *Onchocerciasis,* pp. 14–15.

19. *Ibid.,* pp. 23–36.

20. Waddy, "Control of Onchocerciasis," pp. 851–53; W.H.O. Expert Committee, Second Report, pp. 32–41; Charles Wilcocks and P. E. C. Manson-Bahr, *Manson's Tropical Diseases* (17th ed., London, 1972), p. 228.

21. W.H.O., "Communicable Diseases and Vector Control in 1973," p. 322.

22. J. F. Corson, "The Occurrence of Larvae of *Onchocerca Volvulus* (Leuckart, 1893) in the Skins of Natives of the Gold Coast," *Annals of Tropical Medicine and Parasitology,* XVI (1922), 407–20.

23. A. Fain, "L'Onchocercose dans le bassin du Congo," *Annales de la société belge de médecine tropicale,* LI (1971), 601–3.

24. *Annual Report on the Gold Coast Medical and Sanitary Department,* 1928–29, p. 126; G. F. Saunders, "A Report on Blindness in the Wa and Tumu Districts, Gold Coast, West Africa," *Journal of Tropical Medicine and Hygiene,* XXXVI (1933), 5–6.

25. Budden, "Onchocerciasis in Northern Nigeria," p. 366.

26. Good reviews of the early literature are available in Hoeppli, *Parasitic Diseases,* pp. 136–38, and E. E. Edwards, "Human Onchocerciasis in West Africa with Special Reference to the Gold Coast," *Journal of the West African Science Association,* II (1956), 2–16.

27. *Report of the Ministry of Health,* 1953, p. 100. Several hundred diseases were regularly listed.

28. Medical Report for the Northern Territories, 1907, in *Annual Report on the Northern Territories of the Gold Coast,* 1907, p. 21.

29. Tumu District Record Book, 5–7 August 1912, p. 181, National Archives of Ghana (henceforth NAG) ADM 62/5/1. D.C. signifies District Commissioner; M.O. signifies Medical Officer.

30. Dr. B. B. Waddy to Director of Medical Services, 14 February 1950, Na-

tional Archives of Ghana-Tamale (henceforth NAG-T), Health-34; Director of Medical Services to Waddy, 29 March 1950, NAG-T, Health-34.

31. Tumu District Record Book, "War on Flies," June 1914, p. 233.

32. Principal Medical Officer, Northern Territories, to Principal Medical Officer, Accra, 13 April 1918, NAG ADM 56/1/212.

33. Tumu District Annual Report, 1918, p. 4, NAG ADM 56/1/450.

34. Tumu District Diary, 15–16 April 1917, NAG ADM 66/5/6.

35. *Ibid.*, 2 February 1919, 6 October 1918.

36. *Ibid.*, 29 January 1919.

37. Tumu District Record Book, 28 May 1921, p. 34.

38. *Ibid.*, 1921, p. 4; 1921, p. 36; 1922, p. 86; Tumu District Diary, 10 October 1910, NAG ADM 66/5/6; *ibid.*, 15 November 1916; 25 February 1917; 16 March 1917.

39. The 1911 census was admittedly crude, especially in the north.

40. Lorha [Lawra]-Tumu Official Diary, 14 June 1921, NAG ADM 66/5/7.

41. 1921 census, Lorha-Tumu, p. 5, NAG ADM 56/1/96.

42. Provincial Commissioner Northern Province to Deputy Chief Commissioner Northern Territories, 21 August 1921, NAG ADM 56/1/96.

43. D. C. Navarro to Chief Commissioner Northern Territories (henceforth CCNT), 5 August 1921, NAG ADM 56/1/96. Officials in Wa and Northern Mamprussi failed to comply with requests to compile data on blindness, leprosy, mental derangement, or other disabilities. The 1921 census (NAG ADM 5/2/6) provides an age and sex breakdown by villages, but unfortunately does not give village figures for "infirmities," even for Lorha-Tumu.

44. For example, the Wa District General Information Book (NAG ADM 66/5/2) mentions only two blind chiefs.

45. *Annual Report on the Gold Coast Medical and Sanitary Department, 1928–29*, p. 14. The *Report* for 1930–31 notes that eye diseases were "extremely common" (p. 147).

46. "Report of the Travelling Dispensary," in *Report on the Medical and Sanitary Department, 1928–29*, p. 126.

47. Saunders, "Blindness in Wa and Tumu Districts," p. 5.

48. *Ibid.*, pp. 5–6.

49. M. H. Hughes and P. F. Daly, "Onchocerciasis in the Southern Gold Coast," *Transactions of the Royal Society of Tropical Medicine and Hygiene*, XLV (1951), 243; H. Ridley, *Ocular Onchocerciasis, Including an Investigation of the Gold Coast*, monograph supplement 10, *British Journal of Ophthalmology* (London, 1945), 8.

50. Waddy, "Onchocerciasis and Blindness," p. 3.

51. A. W. Cardinall, *The Gold Coast, 1931* (Accra, 1932), p. 226. This work is the census report for 1931.

52. Lawra-Tumu Diary, 1 June 1934, NAG-T, TNA-1-248. The CCNT minuted: "Good. You have one of the best M.O.s in the Service."

53. *Ibid.*, 26 June 1934 and 9 August 1934.

54. *Ibid.*, 16 August 1934.

55. Annual Report on Navrongo Sub-District of Mamprusi for the Year 1935–36, p. 43, NAG-T, TNA-1-496.

56. Annual Report on Kusasi District, 1932–33, pp. 12–13, NAG-T, TNA-1-543.

57. Bawku Diary, 23 June 1936, NAG ADM 57/5/2. Variant spellings of Wokambo include Wakombo and Waricombo.

58. *Ibid.*, 15 July 1936.

59. *Ibid.*, 16 July 1936.

60. Annual Report on Kusasi District, 1935–36, p. 38, NAG-T, TNA-1-539.

61. Bawku Diary, 13–14 June 1938, NAG ADM 57/5/3 and NAG-T, TNA-1-307.

62. *Ibid.*, 16 June 1938.

63. Bawku Diary, Minutes on 14 and 16 June 1938 entries, NAG-T, TNA-1-307.

64. Annual Report on Kusasi District, 1938–39, p. 23, NAG-T, TNA-1-542.

65. P. Richet, "La Volvulose dans un cercle de la Haute Côte d'Ivoire. Ses Manifestations cutaneés et oculaires," *Bulletin de la société de pathologie exotique*, XXXII (1939), 341–55.

66. NAG, map collection: MP 412, Northwestern Gold Coast, 1905; MP 413, Northeastern Gold Coast, 1905; MP 374, Kusasi, 1938; MP 400, Navrongo, 1928; Hilton, *Population Atlas*, 6, 1931 map.

67. J. K. G. Syme confirms this impression in a personal communication to the author, 15 November 1975.

68. E.g., Tumu District Record Book, p. 155.

69. J. J. Holden, "The Zabarima Conquest of North–West Ghana," *Transactions of the Historical Society of Ghana*, VIII (1965), 60–86.

70. Waddy, "Onchocerciasis and Blindness," p. 8; Hunter, "River Blindness in Nangodi," pp. 410–11.

71. David Scott, *Epidemic Disease in Ghana 1901–1960* (London, 1965), pp. 155–56.

72. *Report on the Medical and Sanitary Department, 1925–26*, Appendix E, "Report on the Incidence of Sleeping Sickness in Lawra District, October, 1924," p. 61.

73. Lawra-Tumu District Annual Report, 1938–39, pp. 39–42, NAG-T, TNA-1-498; *ibid.*, 1939–40, pp. 3, 29–31, NAG-T, TNA-1-506.

74. D.C. Lawra to Medical Officer of Health, Tamale [Waddy], 1 December 1949, NAG-T, Health-34.

75. Assistant Director of Medical Services to CCNT, 7 March 1952, NAG-T, Health-34; Dr. J. W. R. Sarkies, "Report on Blindness and Eye Disease in the Northern Territories of the Gold Coast," NAG-T, Health-34; *Report of the Department of Tsetse Control, 1952–53*, p. 2.

76. Lawra-Tumu Diary, 20 May 1943, NAG ADM 61/5/16.

77. "Conclusions to a Report by K. R. S. Morris and J. H. Hinds," n.d. but c. 1943, NAG-T, Health-34.

78. Waddy, "Onchorcerciasis and Blindness," pp. 35–36. A correlation of -0.29 was found between population growth 1921–48 and blindness. Later, using an exponential curve, he obtained an r = -0.52 (personal communication, 8 September 1975). Waddy erroneously placed population figures for 1921 under a column heading "1931."

79. Saunders, "Report of the Travelling Dispensary," p. 126; "Blindness in Wa and Tumu Districts," p. 5.

80. Ridley, *Ocular Onchocerciasis*, p. 37.

81. M. H. Hughes, "African Onchocerciasis," dissertation for the Degree of Doctor of Medicine, Oxford, 1949, p. 7. Consulted at the Library of the London School of Hygiene and Tropical Medicine.

82. Waddy, "Onchocerciasis and Blindness," p. 10.

83. Hunter, "River Blindness in Nangodi," pp. 414–15; "Seasonal Hunger in a Part of the West African Savanna: A Survey of Bodyweights in North-East Ghana," *Transactions of the Institute of British Geographers*, XLI (1967), 184.

84. Hunter, "River Blindness in Nangodi," pp. 409, 414–15.

85. *Ibid.*, pp. 414–16.

86. Zuarungu District Record Book, II, p. 34, entry for 1935, NAG ADM

68/5/5. Detokko had been occupied for four generations at the time of the interview. It is not clear from the text if "generations" is used as a general indication of time or refers only to the number of chiefs. If the latter is true, settlement might have been somewhat earlier or later.

87. *Ibid.*, p. 79.

88. Navarro [Navrongo] District Record Book, p. 171, NAG ADM 63/5/2.

89. *Ibid.*, p. 247.

90. Zuarungu Diary, 16 June 1917, NAG ADM 68/5/1. Nash attributed this movement to popular confidence in British power to keep the peace and prevent raids.

91. *Ibid.*, 17 June 1917.

92. Zuarungu Diary, 28 October 1913, NAG ADM 68/5/2.

93. Zuarungu Diary, 27 August 1917, NAG ADM 68/5/1.

94. Zuarungu District Record Book, p. 41, NAG ADM 68/5/4.

95. Hilton, "Frafra Resettlement," p. 430; Hunter, "River Blindness in Nangodi," pp. 408–9.

96. Hilton, "Frafra Resettlement," p. 430; Waddy, "Onchocerciasis and Blindness," p. 21; MP 401, Zuarungu, 1946.

97. MP 401; Waddy, "Onchocerciasis and Blindness," pp. 21–22. In some cases farms were still maintained up to within two miles of the river, as at Sekoti and at Tili, opposite Nangodi. See also Hunter, "River Blindness in Nangodi," pp. 408–9; Hilton, "Peuplement de Frafra," pp. 686–87; and Buck, "River Blindness," p. 463.

98. 1931 census, p. 203, NAG ADM 5/2/8.

99. Waddy, "Results of an Investigation into Onchocerciasis and Blindness at Nakong, N.T.s, With Discussion," p. 5, NAG-T, Health-34. Waddy found four former ferrymen at Nangodi; two were blind and one was rapidly losing his sight ("Onchocerciasis and Blindness," p. 22).

100. Informal Diary for Bawku, 25 September 1943, NAG-T, TNA-1-341. The collector was replaced a few days later.

101. *Ibid.*, 29 July 1943. J. K. G. Syme, an observant and experienced D.C., could not recall seeing a visually handicapped ferryman in the many times he used the Nangodi ferry in the 1930s (Personal communication, 15 November 1975). However, there almost certainly were some then.

102. J. K. G. Syme, "The Kusasis: A Short History," pp. 5, 27, 57, 77, unpublished ms., 1932, NAG-T, TNA-1-406; T. E. Hilton, "Notes on the History of Kusasi," *Transactions of the Historical Society of Ghana*, VI (1962), 83–84. Raiding activities are difficult to date, but seem to have been most destructive in the 1860s and 1890s.

103. Syme, "The Kusasis," pp. iv–vi; Hilton, "History of Kusasi," p. 83; Cardinall, *The Gold Coast, 1931*, p. 153.

104. Bawku District Record Book, II, p. 295, NAG ADM 57/5/5; 1931 census, pp. 234–35.

105. Bawku District Record Book, II, p. 304, notation of 17 June 1939; *ibid.*, p. 302.

106. The chief of Wokambo was reportedly going blind in 1923. Bawku District Record Book, I, p. 355, notation of 26 July 1923, NAG ADM 57/5/4.

107. Bawku Diary, 12, 13, 14, 16 June 1938.

108. MP 374; Bawku District Record Book, II, map inserted at p. 312. These ruins may have been of a nineteenth century settlement, but no details are available.

109. 1931 census, pp. 234–35; 1948 census, 342–3, NAG ADM 5/2/9; MP 402, Bawku-Gambaga, 1946.

110. Bawku Diary, 9 March 1936.

111. Bawku District Record Book, II, p. 92.

112. Bawku Diary, 15–16 September 1945, NAG-T, TNA-1-341.

113. Waddy, "Onchocerciasis and Blindness," p. 24.

114. Annual Report on Navrongo Sub-District, 1937–38, p. 22, NAG-T, TNA-1-495; Informal Diary, Navrongo, January 1939–May 1940, 13 February, 24 April, 12 December 1939 and 29 January 1940, NAG ADM 63/5/8; Waddy, "Nakong."

115. Tumu Diary, 24 June 1917; Tumu District Record Book, p. 148, entry for 19–21 March 1917.

116. *Ibid.*, p. 87, entry for Sapari, 17 November 1916; Tumu Diary, 12 November 1916.

117. Hilton, "Settlement Pattern of Tumu," p. 873; Waddy, "Onchocerciasis and Blindness," pp. 35–36.

118. MP 412, 1905.

119. Acting D.C. of Wa to Acting CCNT, 16 June 1910, NAG ADM 56/1/96.

120. M. M. Read, "Essay on the Peoples of the Northwestern Province," pp. 12–13, unpublished ms., 1908, NAG-T, TNA-1-437. Read blamed the ruined villages on Babatu.

121. Hilton, *Population Atlas*, p. 26; Hilton, "Population Growth and Distribution in the Upper Region of Ghana," in John C. Caldwell and Chukuka Okonjo, eds., *The Population of Tropical Africa* (New York, 1968), p. 389. Hilton argues that conditions in Tumu are the culmination of a long process of deterioration linked to river blindness, land abandonment, and soil erosion. Early stages of the process exist in South Mamprusi and intermediate stages in Bawku and Navrongo.

122. F. M. Purcell, "Diet and Nutrition Surveys, Gold Coast. Final Report, 1940," pp. 181–82, NAG ADM 11/1294. The report was published 5 July 1941. Purcell had probably been in contact with Dr. Saunders.

123. *Ibid.*, pp. 26, 83, 86.

124. *Ibid.*, pp. 87, 183.

125. Ridley, *Ocular Onchocerciasis*, p. 8; Waddy, personal communication, 8 September 1975.

126. Ridley, *Ocular Onchocerciasis*, pp. 33–35, 44.

127. Director of Medical Services to Colonial Secretary, 11 June 1945, "Diseases Various: 10 Year Plan," NAG CSO 11/11, 4822.

128. Governor to D.M.S., 26 July 1944, NAG CSO 11/11, 4822; Officer Administering the Government to Secretary of State, 10 September 1946, NAG ADM 1/2/285, no. 270.

129. Waddy, personal communication, 8 September 1975. He was primarily concerned with trypanosomiasis at the time.

130. Waddy, personal communications, 19 October 1975 and 1 January 1976.

131. *Annual Report on the Medical Department, 1947*, p. 1; *ibid.*, 1948, p. 1.

132. Wa District Annual Report, 1947–48, p. 21; NAG-T, TNA-1-537.

133. M. H. Hughes, "Association of Population Changes with Blindness Rates in the Kassena–Nankanni Division of Navrongo District," n.d. but 1948, NAG-T, Health-34; "Depopulation in the Sissili Area," ms., Rhodes House, Oxford, Mss. Afr. S.141, ff. 27–28; "Vare: A Study in Rural Decay," ms., *ibid.*, ff. 29–34. Hughes was unable to continue investigations in the area, but in early 1949 he studied onchocerciasis along the lower Volta in southern Ghana.

134. Waddy, "A Report on an Onchocerciasis Survey Held at Tili," 1948, NAG-T, Health-34.

135. Waddy, "Nakong," pp. 1–3.

136. *Ibid.,* p. 4.

137. *Ibid.,* p. 5.

138. Waddy to Health Department, Tamale, 25 May 1948, NAG-T, Health-34.

139. Waddy, personal communication, 8 September 1975.

140. Waddy, "Onchocerciasis and Blindness," *passim.*

141. The Medical Department wanted to publish it, but the Government Printer was too busy. Government Printer to D.M.S. Accra, 15 December 1950, NAG-T, Health-34.

142. R. Puyuelo and M. M. Holstein, "L'Onchocercose humaine en Afrique noire française: maladie sociale," *Médecine Tropicale,* X (1950), 397–510.

143. Puyuelo to Waddy, 23 January 1950; Waddy to Puyuelo, 27 March, 1950; NAG-T, Health-34. Neither Waddy nor Ridley had been aware of French work. Although Ridley does list Richet's 1938 paper in his bibliography, he neither cites it in this text nor indicates that he was aware of its contents. He probably saw only the uninformative 3-line abstract in *Tropical Diseases Bulletin,* CCCLXXVI (1940), 100. See also Waddy, "Frontiers and Disease in West Africa," *Journal of Tropical Medicine and Hygiene,* LXI (1958), 100–107.

144. *Annual Report on the Medical Department, 1951,* p. 13.

145. Rodger, *Blindness in West Africa,* p. 34.

146. Sarkies, "Report on Blindness and Eye Disease," p. 2.

147. *Annual Report on the Medical Department, 1952,* p. 9. The studies were published as Rodger, *Blindness in West Africa,* and Crisp, *Simulium and Onchocerciasis.*

148. Official census figures were about 407,000 in 1921 and 736,000 in 1948.

149. W.H.O. Expert Committee, Second Report, p. 11; Crisp, *Simulium and Blindness,* p. 42. For recent examples, see Knüttgen, "Onchocerciasis in Upper Guinea," p. 611; and J. Lagraulet, "Epidemiology of Ocular Onchocerciasis in French-Speaking Countries of West Africa," *Israeli Journal of Medical Science,* VIII (1972), 1153.

150. Crisp, *Simulium and Onchocerciasis,* p. 49.

151. Bawku Diary, 24 June 1936 and 1 March 1937, NAG ADM 57/5/2.

152. B. B. Waddy, "Some Reminiscences of the Western Northern Territories of the Gold Coast," *The Nigerian Field,* XXII (1957), 84.

153. Waddy, personal communication, 1 January 1976. Every M.O. had access to current literature, because the Medical Department distributed *Tropical Diseases Bulletin* and the *Bulletin of Hygiene* to them.

154. For a recent example, see Buck, "River Blindness," p. 457.

155. Waddy, "Frontiers and Disease," p. 106.

156. Budden, "Onchocerciasis in Northern Nigeria," pp. 366–67.

157. *Report of the Ministry of Health, 1954,* p. 46. See also Scott, *Epidemic Disease in Ghana,* p. ix. The author of this chapter is working on a general study of colonial medicine in the region.

5

Epidemic Disease Among the Sara
of Southern Chad, 1890–1940

Mario Joaquim Azevedo

Around the world, conquest and subsequent colonialism increased communication and thus introduced new diseases or helped spread those that were endemic or sporadic. Smallpox and other diseases, which killed thousands of Amerindians, came in with the Spanish conquistadores.[1] The same thing occurred among the Tasmanians and New Guineans.[2] William Peterson notes that: "Europeans have transported . . . to other parts of the world syphilis, malaria, tuberculosis, measles, whooping cough, chicken pox, dysentery, smallpox, and even the common cold; and all of those were more often fatal among the new hosts than in Europe."[3]

In Africa long-distance trade and the advent of colonialism created circumstances that favored the spread of infectious diseases. Philip Curtin has echoed this thesis: "In the longer sweep of history . . . increased intercommunication has made disease environments more nearly alike, not more diverse; but each breach of previous isolation has brought higher death rates, as unfamiliar diseases attacked populations whose environment provided no source of immunity."[4] Sleeping sickness (trypanosomiasis), venereal diseases, smallpox, malaria, and cerebrospinal meningitis are examples of diseases that accompanied the breakdown of barriers between previously isolated peoples. In this sense colonialism indirectly contributed to a rise in death rate among Africans.

Epidemics killing thousands were common in Chad at the end of the nineteenth century and during the first half of the twenti-

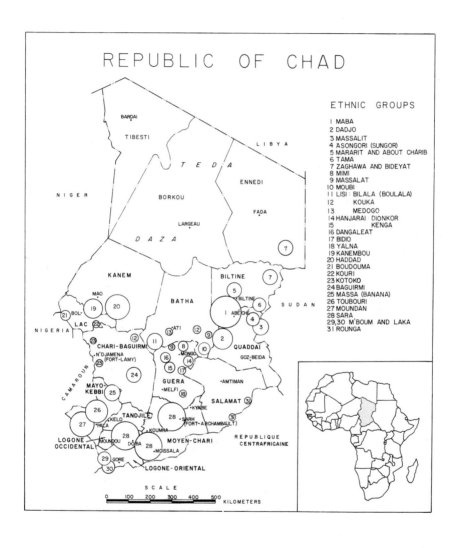

REPUBLIC OF CHAD

BARDAI

TIBESTI

LIBYA

T E D A

ENNEDI

NIGER

BORKOU

FADA

LARGEAU

D A Z A

KANEM

MAO

BATHA

BILTINE

19   20

BOL·

NIGERIA

LAC   22

CHARI-BAGUIRMI

12

N'DJAMENA
(FORT-LAMY)

CAMAROUN

23

MAYO-
KEBBI

25

26

TANDJILE

27   PALA   KELO

LOGONE
OCCIDENTAL   MOUNDOU   DOBA

29   GORE

30

LOGONE-ORIENTAL

GUERA

24   MELFI

BILTINE   7

5   BILTINE

ABECHE   6

1   4   3

ATI   12

13   9   2

11   9   8   10   QUADDAI

16   MONGO   GOZ-BEIDA

15   14

17

18

AMTIMAN

SALAMAT

KYABE   31

28   SARH   31
(FORT-ARCHAMBAULT)

KOUMRA

28   MOYEN-CHARI

28   MOISSALA

SUDAN

REPUBLIQUE
CENTRAFRICAINE

ETHNIC GROUPS

1 MABA
2 DADJO
3 MASSALIT
4 ASONGORI (SUNGOR)
5 MARARIT AND ABOUT CHARIB
6 TAMA
7 ZAGHAWA AND BIDEYAT
8 MIMI
9 MASSALAT
10 MOUBI
11 LISI: BILALA (BOULALA)
12   KOUKA
13   MEDOGO
14 HANJARAI: DIONKOR
15   KENGA
16 DANGALEAT
17 BIDIO
18 YALNA
19 KANEMBOU
20 HADDAD
21 BOUDOUMA
22 KOURI
23 KOTOKO
24 BAGUIRMI
25 MASSA (BANANA)
26 TOUBOURI
27 MOUNDAN
28 SARA
29,30 M'BOUM AND LAKA
31 ROUNGA

SCALE

0   100   200   300   400   500
                              KILOMETERS

eth. The major contention of this study is that intercommunication and physical mobility, increased greatly by the French
presence, inadvertently fostered epidemics, and thus increased
mortality from diseases in Chad. The spread of epidemics coincided with altered patterns of intercommunication during the
early colonial period. Explorers and travelers such as Heinrich
Barth and Casimir Maistre did not mention any epidemics while
visiting Chad during the nineteenth century. One must assume
that serious epidemic diseases were not alarming enough to attract the visitors' attention or that of their African informants.
But Europeans were not solely responsible for the spread of disease; Arab and African traders also share the responsibility. What
the European presence did, however, was to accelerate a process
that otherwise might have taken centuries. The end result was
severe demographic instability in all Sara districts of southern
Chad and depopulation in specific areas.

French administrators consistently singled out disease as the
major cause of demographic instability and depopulation in
French Equatorial Africa. The merit of this hypothesis will be
analyzed in this study which is based on archival material in
N'Djamena (Chad) and Paris and on oral data collected among
the Sara of Chad in 1974.[5] The focus is on specific major epidemics that affected southern Chad, including sleeping sickness,
cerebrospinal meningitis, smallpox, venereal diseases, and the
"Spanish" influenza pandemic of 1918.

Sleeping Sickness

Sleeping sickness apparently caused a higher death toll than
other epidemic diseases. The disease is caused by parasitic protozoa called trypanosomes which attack both men and domesti-
cated animals. The parasites are transmitted from one host to
another by species of tsetse fly of the genus Glossina, such as *G.
palpalis* or *G. tachinoides*. The favorite habitat of *G. tachinoides*
is the dry savannah woodland along river banks and lakes with
green vegetation. *G. palpalis* prefers the tropical rain forest with

its moister environment. The worst ravages occur in the dry savannah lands; as a whole they are actually less infested by the
tsetse fly, but because both man and fly are looking for the scarce
water, they are more likely to come into contact with one another.[6] Once a fly carries the trypanosome, it will continue to do
so for the rest of its life. McKelvey describes the symptoms of
the disease:

> It starts wth a simple red swelling at the site of a tsetse bite.
> Malaise, lassitude, and low-grade fever lasting off and on for two years
> may ensue. Insomnia at night, drowsiness during the daytime, and
> headache constitute some of the observable symptoms. Soon after the
> onset of the disease a rash may appear, especially around the trunk,
> chest, and back; . . . muscular cramps and neurological pains become
> common. Swollen glands are another sign.[7]

Then the patient begins to lose his memory and tends to doze
while sitting or eating. Frequent periods of sleepiness soon progress into a coma. The patient loses his appetite and his ability
to control urinary and bowel functions. Sometimes the patient
may recover briefly, but eventually dies from pneumonia-like
complications.[8]

Present evidence suggests that African trypanosomiasis began
in West Africa and eventually spread to East Africa. K. R. S.
Morris observes that it probably existed on the Upper Niger during the fourteenth century since its symptoms were mentioned by
the Arab historian, Ibn Khaldun. The king of Mali, Mansa Djata,
reportedly died from it in 1374.[9] R. Hoeppli noted that sleeping
sickness was mentioned by Arab writers in the fourteenth century, by John Atkins along the Guinea Coast in 1721, and by
observers in Sierra Leone in 1803, and again during the 1840s.
These early reports refer only to West Africa, not to Central
Africa.[10] We are not sure whether the disease existed in Equatorial Africa before the turn of the twentieth century when
French authorities initially reported it. Morris contends that at
the end of the nineteenth century the disease had reached the
Congo Basin from West Africa, where it had been endemic during the previous century. It spread along the Congo's elaborate
tributary system between 1885 and 1896. Thus, "when the French

occupied their Equatorial African colony in 1890, the disease was already present on the Ubangi River, the great northern affluent of the Congo." Between 1890 and 1906 it reached the Nile in Uganda and then entered southern Sudan. "Thus," Morris continues, "epidemics in the interior of the Congo reached their height in 1906–20, two decades earlier than occurred in the West African hinterland, lacking river communications."[11] The spread of the disease was furthered during the 1880s and 90s by the Madhist movement in Sudan, by the caravans of men like Tippu-Tib, a Zanzibari ivory trader, and by Belgian and Arab traders.[12] In the 1920s its presence was general in western, central, eastern, and southern Africa.

Morris offers the following description of the entry of the disease into Chad.

> Significantly, the extension of the disease followed the old caravan route which had been adopted by the French in 1901 for linking the Ubangui and Chad. . . . By the middle of 1915, however, the epidemic had developed to such a height that, during the following two years it killed so many people that the survivors could no longer bury their dead. The attempts to flee from infected villages spread the disease from place to place so widely that, within a few years, the whole network of rivers comprising the Chari basin was involved in the epidemic.[13]

The most favorable habitat for the tsetse fly in Chad lies along river banks in Sara country. Once *Trypanosoma gambiensie* infects the vectors in a district, it tends to remain unless it is intentionally eradicated or the climate changes radically. The destructiveness of sleeping sickness in the first twenty years of our century is difficult to comprehend. In some areas of Chad, such as Fort-Lamy, Moissala, Gorée, and Moundou, the disease infected over 55 percent of the population, almost decimating entire villages, frequently forcing the survivors to search for safer places.[14] Until 1950 trypanosomiasis was common in the prefectures of Moyen-Chari (Fort-Archambault), the two Logones (with centers at Moundou and Doba), and Chari-Baguirmi (even at Fort-Lamy).[15] Its social effects are awesome. R. Kuczynski, writing in 1939 about the Cameroons and Togoland, observed that "sleeping sickness is a powerful anticonceptional factor" and that "under its influence the number of deaths exceeds that of births in all epidemics and endemo-epidemic foci."[16]

The archival material, as shown in Table 1, simply mentions the gravity and frequency of sleeping sickness, which was known as *bir* or *mey-bi* among the Sara. It does not present complete reports that would enable one to determine even an approximate number of people who were either infected with the disease or who perished from it. Fortunately Father Alcantara's accounts in addition to the oral narratives of Sara elders give us an impression of the severe ravages of the epidemic. Several Catholic missionaries, for example, succumbed to the disease.

Table 1. *Trypanosomiasis in Chad (1890–1940)*

Year	Region	Number of sick	Number of deaths
1912	Filtri	—	—
1920	Moyen-Logone	—	—
	Guira Village	—	150
1922	Moyen-Logone	—	—
	Moyen-Chari	—	—
1925	Moyen-Logone	—	—
	Moyen-Chari	—	"several thousands"
1930	Fort-Lamy area	28	—
1931–1943	Moundou, Doba and vicinity	—	"thousands of victims"
1934	Moyen-Chari	3,608	—
	Fort-Archambault	14	—
	Kemassa	365–380	—
	Guire	—	10
	Dai	7	—
1937	Moissala and Koumra	650	—
1940	Doba	515	143 (27 percent of sick)

Sources: W90, 11–17, 1912, p. 8; W19, 5, 1920, p. 20; W1, 10, 1922, (n.p.); W1, 15, 1925, p. 4; W19, (n.n.), 1930, (n.p.); Pierre d'Alcantara, "La maladie du sommeil," in *Le Courier du Logone—Nouvelles du Diocèse de Moundou.* Tchad, 55 (1971), 3 ff; W37, 6, 1937, p. 70; W29, 9, 1940, (n.p.).

Oral information from areas struck by the disease prior to 1970 reveal the human suffering it caused in Chad, especially in the relatively densely populated areas of Sara districts. Three men from the village of Kou, about 65 kilometers from Doba, described what happened to their village in the 1930s and why only 74 persons lived there in 1974. Kou was nothing more than a forest until the Fathers of the Holy Spirit opened a mission there in April 1929. Hundreds of people gathered around Kou and it grew rapidly. In less than two years 24 marriages, 153 baptisms, and 88 confirmations had been performed.[17] Several things attracted people to the new center: the kindness of the missionaries, particularly their Superior, Father Herriau; sufficient well-water; and perhaps more importantly, tax collection. The missionaries themselves collected the taxes from all Kou residents and took the receipts to the authorities at Doba or Moundou, thus preventing abuses.[18]

Furthermore, every Kou inhabitant was exempt from forced labor. In a few years the mission extended itself over six miles in each direction. It appears from oral information that approximately a thousand people came within its sphere. The settlement naturally alarmed the neighboring chief as well as the administrator of Doba. Both were losing control over their subjects as the missionaries' prestige increased. But the mission and Kou experienced a terrible setback when a sleeping sickness epidemic erupted.

> In a few months the tsetse flies invaded the mission, infected animals and people, the livestock of the mission was annihilated; . . . children fell sick and died . . . Father Weiss and Rev. Denis, a religious Brother, returned to France, seriously ill.[19]

A few months later the Superior, Father Herriau, suddenly returned to France for treatment of sleeping sickness. In 1932 the French authorities forced the Holy Spirit missionaries to close the mission at Kou, now considered a center for the dissemination of the disease. Everyone vacated Kou under governmental orders. The old bricks of the chapel and the trees planted by Father Herriau are the surviving monuments of the mission effort. Father Alcantara believes that no less than two-thirds of the people living near rivers died from the disease by 1935.[20]

In Moissala and its surrounding areas along the Barh Sara River, the death toll, especially during the 1920s, was likewise very high.[21] In 1924 the disease struck Moyonogo, a community with some five thousand people, taking hundreds to their graves. People moved to Bidja and Beili in Oubangui-Chari (Central African Empire). The people of Guira, stricken by the epidemic, subsequently moved to the village of Morko to receive treatment. The village of Silambi also suffered from the epidemic; its chief was among those who perished. From Silambi the disease spread to Koumra, Dagre, Bedjondo, Gabian, and the canton of Modele. People deserted the villages of Mayngama and Ngendoumou.

The administration created a special center at Morolo to receive the people. Doctors compelled some people from the canton of Bedeke to settle at the newly created village, which soon received the name of Mousnini. People went to Mousnini to be cured, but in most cases they died there. Literally, Mousnini means "bury the dead here," or "the place of the dead," the cemetery. Mousnini today has over 500 dwellers. The village of Gabian, which numbered some 2,500 people in 1924, now has about 250. At Mousnini informants reported that at least three out of every ten villagers died from the disease. Since preventive medical services and aid arrived only after the outbreak of the epidemic, the majority of those stricken died.[22]

At Bodo, near Doba, a similar account was given in detail by Father Réné, a Capuchin missionary in his seventies, who witnessed some of the epidemics in Oubangui-Chari. He reported that it was common to see three out of ten people die. At the Moundou hospital so many died that the bodies could not be buried quickly enough. The old missionary concluded by saying that if a "cure" had not been found, the whole Sara population in Bodo would have disappeared during the 1930s. "They died like flies," he said.[23] Five kilometers from Doba lies Beraba, a village which became a refuge for patients awaiting treatment. Scores of sick came from Bebedja, Miandoum, Mongo, Damala,

Gorée, and other places. At least six-tenths of the new arrivals died before or shortly after their treatment started. The villagers resented their presence because they did not care to bury people they did not know.[24]

It is curious, as D. Scott points out, that "in general Gambian sleeping sickness is a disease of males rather than of females, and of the working age group of men in particular."[25] Under endemic conditions the proportion of sick men to sick women is two to one. When epidemics occur, however, the gap closes. The reason for the difference under endemic conditions is that working age men typically traveled more than women or may have fished for hours on tsetse-infested rivers.

What effect did the epidemic have on the fertility of women? As yet there is no conclusive evidence. A recent study of infertility in tropical Africa by Anne Retel-Laurentin notes that "sleeping sickness cannot be considered responsible for sterility. . . . However, one can assume that fertility decreased during the period of the epidemics because of the transitory sterilizing injuries which occur at the septicemic phase of the disease; indeed, permanent sterility was observed among people whose treatment was late."[26]

The first fight for the eradication of the disease in French Equatorial Africa including Chad was led by Drs. Albert Schweitzer and Eugéne Jamot. Jamot left France shortly before 1914 to work with the Institut Pasteur at Brazzaville. Schweitzer spent his time at Lambarène, Gabon, near the Ogooué River. Jamot, on the other hand, traveled all over French Equatorial Africa and as far as Upper Volta. Both men used atoxyl from 1916 to 1918, but thereafter gave tryparsamide to treat sleeping sickness. Both drugs helped patients; but in some unfortunate cases overdoses of the drugs caused permanent blindness.[27] Alcantara mentions that even moranyl, a serum extracted from horses and used until 1942, could cause blindness.[28]

The final question concerns responsibility for the spread of the disease and its change from endemicity to epidemicity. Few who have studied the disease doubt that the French must assume most of this responsibility. By increasing mobility and contact between distant localities, they helped carry the vector. Had they combined economic and communication activities with available health services, the cost in suffering and death might not have been as high. Morris notes the role in spreading the disease played by soldiers, laborers, and Arab traders "employed by the Belgian and the French in opening up their newly acquired Central African territories."[29] Before the European arrival in the interior of central Africa, trade was localized and organized in such a way that one ethnic group transported its goods to the limits of its district, and the next group did the same. Under these conditions, numerous diseases could remain endemic indefinitely. European activities changed that. "The needs of colonization intensified considerably and enlarged the circuits of exchange. The perpetual displacement of men, long-distance portage, and river transportation in Central Africa, bear the responsibility for the continuous and rapid progress of the epidemic."[30] John McKelvey notes that "European development had unwittingly made it possible for native and imported diseases to ravage human populations and their animals. This European influence, in large part intended to do the African people good, presented on its other face a curse."[31]

It is apparent that sleeping sickness existed in West Africa before the arrival of the Europeans, but in an endemic form. At the end of the nineteenth century, increased contacts between people helped spread the disease, and transformed it into a recurrent epidemic. The greater use of rivers, some of which had been infested by the tsetse fly, also favored disease dissemination. Both changes were encouraged by Europeans after the partition of the continent. By 1912 the inhabitants of Central Africa, including the southern half of Chad, suffered from epidemic trypanosomiasis.

The incomplete nature of the archival material does not allow us to enumerate the casualties caused by the dreaded disease in Chad as a whole or among the Sara. There are no statistics to indicate how many Chadians lived along the rivers before 1940. But this much is clear: the most severely infected places in Chad were Doba, Moissala, Moundou, and Sarh. In the words of Retel-

Laurentin, "millions got the disease and thousands died from it."[32] Depopulation in the strict sense no doubt occurred in these districts before 1940. The consensus is that approximately one-third of the riverine people in Chad perished during the recurrent epidemics of sleeping sickness. The inhabitants of Moyen-Chari and the two Logones were especially hard hit.

Cerebrospinal Meningitis

Cerebrospinal meningitis, like sleeping sickness, was responsible for the death of thousands of Chadians, particularly after 1890. Interviewed elders recall clearly that meningitis existed in Chad before Europeans arrived. They cannot understand, however, why in the first decades of the century it seemed to become more prevalent, causing an unusually high number of deaths. Colonial reports are often silent about endemic diseases but speak out whenever health conditions change dramatically.

Cerebrospinal meningitis is caused by a bacterium, *Neisseria meningitidis*, which infects the respiratory passages. After two to five days of incubation, "the illness starts suddenly with a rigor and fever, a severe headache and vomiting; convulsions are common in children."[33] Bleeding, collapse, and vomiting are signs of imminent death. If the patient recovers, he may become deaf or "mentally deficient." Since the 1940s, treatment with sulphonamides and antibiotics has been effective. It is a seasonal disease, occurring during the dry months between January and May. In Africa its favorite habitat is the dry region between the Sahara desert and the equatorial forest, in countries such as Chad, northern Nigeria, and Upper Volta, where out of the tens of thousands of people who are stricken annually, some 12 percent die.[34]

The mobility created by colonial administrations in West and Central Africa enhanced the spread of this disease over larger areas. Several meningitis epidemics occurred in Chad; they undoubtedly contributed to demographic loss. B. B. Waddy's studies show that epidemics spread from "east to west in Africa, north of the Equator and south of the Sahara." He traces the disease's relentless movement from Sudan to Senegal.[35] In the late 1920s and early 1930s meningitis was present among the population of central Sudan. Then it moved westward to Wadai in eastern Chad, passing along the major caravan and pilgrim route. In 1937 it reached southeastern Chad, Lake Chad, and Nigeria. It then continued westward through Niger and Ghana; by 1941 it had spread as far west as Sierra Leone and the Senegambia area. Waddy notes, however, that "it must be admitted that CSM had been present in French Equatorial Africa before this [1935]. From 1932 to 1935 there were small epidemics localized round Mayo Kebbi [Chad] in the West."[36] Archival material, in fact, suggests the existence of limited epidemics even in the 1910s.[37]

The worst epidemic disaster on record in Chad occurred in 1938. According to an army doctor, Colonel Ledentu, Inspector-General of Health and Medical Services of French Equatorial Africa, mortality was so great in virtually all of Chad, particularly in Sara country, that the authorities of Logone (Moundou and Doba) complained of a scarcity of manpower. Doba alone counted 1,008 deaths in the first half of the year.[38] According to Ledentu, the epidemic began in the first half of 1937 at the crossroads between Fort-Archambault and Am-Timan, to the east; at the same time it appeared north of Moundou, to the west. It moved swiftly to Fort-Lamy, Koumra, Boda, Lère, and Bouzoum; next it spread north to Mao, near Lake Chad and south to the border of Lobaye (subdivision of Carnot); then it mercilessly ravaged Haute-Sanga, Ouahm, Mayo-Kebbi, and Baguirmi.[39] Colonel Ledentu's chart (Table 2) gives us some idea of its death toll during that year.

Most deaths, about 1,660, occurred in the Sara prefectures of Logone and Moyen-Chari. The subprefectures most affected were Koumra, Moissala, and Doba, with a total of 1,345 deaths, "over one-third of the total number of victims of the epidemic of 1938."[40] Over 95 percent of the inhabitants of these subprefectures are Sara. Ledentu broke down the statistics of 78 deaths according to age and sex and remarked that the epidemic struck young adults and children particularly hard, except in Haute-Sanga where older adults were stricken as well.[41] Taking into

Table 2. *Cerebrospinal Meningitis Epidemic, 1936–37*

Department	Subdivision	Duration of epidemic	Cases reported	Deaths recorded
Haute-Sanga (C.A. Emp.)	Carnot	Nov. 30–Feb. 24		89
Kemo-Gribingui (C.A. Emp.)	Crampel	End of Dec.–Jan. 11		19
Bas-Chari	Massakory	Jan. 1–Mar. 15	320	298
	Fort-Lamy	Mar. 13–May 3	252	201
	Rural Areas			100
Logone	Moundou	Jan. 15–April	182	145
	Lai	Feb. 14–Mar. 4	32	20
	Baibokoum	Feb. 22–April	150	150
	Doba	Feb. 15–Apr. 30	744	645
Moyen-Chari	Koumra	Jan. 15–April	295	701
	Moissala	Feb.–April	52	
Kanem		Jan.–Apr. 15		211
Baguirmi	Melfi	Feb. 3–Apr. 18		40
	Mousso	Feb.–Apr.		369
	Massenya	Mar. 18–Apr. 7		3
Ouahm	Batangafo	Feb. 14–Apr.		89
Mayo Kebbi	Palla	Mar.–Apr.		156
	Fianga	Mar.–Apr.		12
	Bangor			12
Salamat		Apr. 6–Apr. 8		2
Total				3,262

consideration unreported cases, he estimated that at least 5,000 people died in Chad in 1938, or about 0.4 percent of the inhabitants of the colony in that year. The number of deaths at Doba represents approximately 3 percent of the population in the Sara subdivision—enough in itself to prevent any population growth for that year.[42]

Clearly then, the number of recorded deaths increased as the years passed, despite the slow improvement of medical care. The situation had not drastically changed by 1951. From 1943 to 1951 deaths from the disease may have kept the death rate in Chad (4 percent per year) close to the birth rate for that period (4.15 percent).[43] The number of deaths caused by meningitis was certainly not enough to create depopulation, but the demographic picture is sobering when one is aware that sleeping sickness was also present in the same districts.

Smallpox

In some years smallpox was as deadly as meningitis and sleeping sickness in Chad. The degree to which smallpox was present in former French Equatorial Africa before the end of the nineteenth century is still unclear. Sara elders assumed that the disease was endemic in southern Chad before the arrival of the French. For central and northern Chad in particular, the trans-Saharan trade route and the east/west pilgrimage route may have provided opportunities for repeated introduction of the disease.

Colonial reports of the twentieth century lament the recurrence of smallpox; in 1922, for example, there was a severe outbreak in Moissala.[44] Another epidemic erupted among Sara school children in February and March 1924, brought in from Fort-Lamy by a serviceman's wife, killing six children. The most serious epidemic occurred in 1925 when the prefecture of Moyen-Chari registered 30,000 smallpox patients, of whom 6,000 died. The deaths represented approximately 20 percent of the patients and about 3.3 percent of the entire population of Moyen-Chari, then estimated at 180,000. In the subdivision of Pala there was another outbreak in 1929, but the death toll was not recorded.[45] Three years later another local epidemic appeared northeast of Fort-Lamy, in the subdivision of N'Gaur. Fifty-two persons reportedly contracted the disease with only eight recorded deaths. Some measures were taken to prevent its spread: officials closed the markets of Mallum and Kuludia, isolated persons, vaccinated 6,107 people, and halted travelers attempting to enter Chad from Nigeria and the Cameroon, since the disease apparently came from those countries.[46]

Compared to sleeping sickness, smallpox was seemingly less frequent in Chad. Its demographic impact, with the exception of the 1925 epidemic, may not have been as harmful as that of sleeping sickness. Moreover, sleeping sickness was normally confined to dry areas where water was available, and along river banks, whereas smallpox simply accompanied people. Thus, when medical services were available, it was easier to check the spread of smallpox. But smallpox had a serious side effect; it frequently induced abortion among pregnant women.[47] As a result, it may have had an adverse impact on birth rates in the affected districts. In relation to meningitis, official records do not reveal which of the two claimed more victims before 1940, but if the deaths of 1938 indicate the severity of cerebrospinal meningitis, then we can conclude that it caused higher mortality rates than smallpox.

Venereal Disease

Doctors and epidemiologists continue to wrestle with the problems of venereal diseases, which are currently spreading at an alarming rate in developing countries. The Chadian government is very concerned about this problem, especially among secondary school students in urban centers. Earlier colonial administrators bemoaned the same condition. To the elders, widespread venereal diseases are a direct result of lax morality caused by modernization. Table 3, based upon Stephen Reyna's study, gives an idea of the seriousness of the present situation in Chad. As Reyna points out, the number of infected people among the Muslims of Chad was almost double that of non-Muslim people in 1970; at least one percent of the total population of the territory was reportedly affected.[48] Because such diseases may be a cause of female sterility in Equatorial Africa, they deserve attention as an important demographic variable.

Syphilis is caused by a spirochete known as *Treponema pallidum* and is transmitted primarily through sexual intercourse. Gonorrhea, caused by *Neisseria gonorrhoeae,* seems to induce a

Table 3. *Distribution of Venereal Diseases in Chad, 1970*

	Muslim	Non-Muslim	Not identified by region	Chari-Baguirmi (a Sara prefecture)	Total
Syphilis	5,644	533	4,041	1,823	10,218
Gonorrhea	11,186	6,291	5,664	4,753	23,141
Total venereal diseases	16,850	6,824	9,705	6,576	33,379
Total number of inhabitants	1,325,588	1,611,246		347,666	2,936,834
Percent infected	1.3	0.4		1.9	

loss of fertility, but the actual process of sterilization is not yet adequately understood.[49] The following discussion is based on recent works by Retel-Laurentin and Anatole Romaniuk studying the impact of venereal diseases on fertility among tropical populations in Africa.[50]

The origins of venereal diseases among the Sara are not certain. Most Sara elders interviewed are convinced that either the French or the Arabs introduced venereal diseases, especially syphilis and gonorrhea. They identified French soldiers in Chad as the major carriers. A chief of *carré* in Koumra naively but seriously contended that French dogs were the original carriers of venereal diseases. He argued that French widows trained their dogs sexually, contracted syphilis and gonorrhea, and in turn transmitted them to men, particularly soldiers, who constantly sought women for sexual gratification. The soldiers then became the long-distance carriers of the disease. "This is how these diseases appeared in Chad; the French soldiers introduced them here," he added.[51] Elders of Bouna reportedly saw the disease for the first time in 1942 when they returned from Fort-Archambault. Elderly women from the village of Kol (near Koumra) still remember Sunamta, the woman who first contracted the disease in their village in the early 1920s.[52] Elsewhere villagers related that when the disease first appeared in the late nineteenth century, a victim was completely isolated from the community. Food, clothes, drinks, and medicines were virtually thrown at the victim to avoid physical contact. As the years passed, the disease became so widespread that it was impractical to isolate the infected. Educated Chadians, including doctors, gave essentially the same opinion as their grandfathers when interviewed.

The French community, however, is divided. Laymen tend to uphold the opinion that venereal diseases appeared long before the French arrival. While some French missionaries suspect that the Sara elders are right, others think that Arabs originally introduced venereal diseases and that the French simply aggravated the situation.[53] Romaniuk is convinced that the European presence in the nineteenth century encouraged the spread of venereal diseases in Equatorial Africa. Retel-Laurentin agrees more with the oral data of elders as well as some reports of European explorers and writers. Without explicitly saying that venereal disease was not there before, she claims that a diffusion took place between 1895 and 1914. Syphilis was first reported in Gabon and the Congo River mouth. In Kasai it was identified in 1896. Soon it appeared to spread up the Congo River and its confluents to Sangha (Central African Empire), Sankuru, Chuwapa, and Lomela (in Zaire). Further north the Bahr-el-Ghazal and the Nile caravan routes no doubt helped to diffuse venereal disease into Central Africa. So between 1900 and 1910, syphilis and gonorrhea became more common in some Chadian communities.[54] E. H. Hudson, however, postulated that the organism causing syphilis originated in Equatorial Africa. He argued that the disease could change from one form to another depending on the environment and man's social history, without a mutation on the part of the bacterium itself. He pointed out that Central Africa, because of its heat and humidity "in historic times," was the most probable first habitat of the *Treponema pallidum*. He wrote:

The thesis here advanced suggests that treponemal infection of man originated in Equatorial Africa as yaws, in Paleolithic times, that it accompanied the hunter-gatherers in their migrations, and that it changed to endemic syphilis in cooler and drier areas. Endemic syphilis found an exceptionally favorable environment in the village, a social invention of Mesolithic/Neolithic time which spread over the world, the New as well as the Old.[55]

In his opinion, syphilis is an urban disease, and it evolved in the Middle East for the first time because of the new social conditions, where ". . . coitus in practical terms became the only personal contact of sufficient intimacy to permit transmission of treponemes." Hudson's hypothesis has been rejected by many writers who consider the supporting evidence weak.[56]

But the critical questions are whether or not syphilis and gonorrhea became sufficiently common to decrease the population after 1890 and what kind of specific impact the diseases had on fertility among the Chadian Sara. A report filed in 1910 from Fort-Archambault complains of the spread of these diseases. In 1922, 50 cases had been registered in the small "hospital" of

Fort-Archambault.[57] The administrator of colonies, Georges Bruel, mentioned in 1918 the seriousness of the situation in Equatorial Africa and blamed the soldiers, guards, and workers, for their expansion.[58] Another report notes that syphilis and gonorrhea were the most widespread diseases in the prefecture of Moyen-Chari.[59] It is unfortunate that no statistical information accompanied this report.

There are a few figures for Chari-Baguirmi prefecture. The prefecture's reports of 1931, 1932, 1934, and 1935, studied by Reyna, called the disease "le fleau du pays," (the scourge of the country). In 1935, 245 blood tests were taken at Fort-Lamy and 27 cases were detected; that is, 11 percent of the examined patients. During the same year, the capital, with a total population of 4,000 people, had approximately 320 prostitutes. They were tested for gonorrhea, and 49 percent of the 288 prostitutes examined had positive signs.[60] Opinions differ on the significance of venereal diseases as a cause of sterility. Retel-Laurentin notes that from 1900 to 1930 Europeans linked tropical sterility to venereal diseases, and similarly both Romaniuk and Retel-Laurentin continue to argue for the possibility of a cause and effect relationship. Retel-Laurentin has found that in at least two-thirds of the women infected by gonorrhea there is sterility or very low fertility. The puzzle is that the remaining one-third remain fertile.[61]

Clarification of the word fertility as used by demographers is important at this point. Fertility for a given population is considered normal if the number of births allows the population to grow. In Retel-Laurentin's opinion, for fertility to be normal in sub-Saharan Africa, each woman must have an average of four children during her reproductive life. When venereal disease has reached 50 percent of a population, the average number of children per woman does not exceed two; if this "index of syphilis" is 30 to 40 percent, the average will be three to four children; if less than 10 percent, then its impact on overall fertility is negligible.[62] Again, the nature of archival material does not indicate the numerical extent of the disease in the south. Although the south has a higher birth rate than the north, its mortality rate is also higher and its life expectancy lower.[63]

We have interesting studies of the population of the Sorko canton in the subdivision of Melfi (700 kilometers east of N'Djamena, formerly Fort-Lamy) by two military doctors, Moulinard (April–May 1935), and Lauret (May 1936).[64] The population of Melfi was given as 60,602 in 1924; by 1931 it had dropped to 42,133. Moulinard found that birth rates had declined and that mortality had increased since 1924. He interviewed 33 women who claimed to have had a total of 150 pregnancies, which resulted in 26 abortions, 72 dead infants (including still-births), and 52 living babies. Such results gave a 3.75–4.50 fertility rate (or "index of general capacity"). He further claimed that for a community of 4,325, he registered 282 deaths and 180 births for a twelve-month period without serious epidemics. Comparing the year 1924 with 1931, the doctor noted that for 38,357 adults in 1924 there were 22,245 children (36 percent of the total population), whereas in 1931, for 29,872 adults he registered only 12,261 children, that is, down to 29 percent of the population. He attributed the decline to psychological and social disturbances accompanying colonialism. Could venereal diseases have been a factor also? Perhaps.

Alarmed by Moulinard's report, Dr. Lauret arrived in 1936 to verify the facts *in loco*. Lauret came up with a higher birth rate and a lower mortality rate. Moulinard's 6.52 percent mortality contrasted with 4.74 percent by Lauret. The total population declined by 36 percent according to Moulinard, but increased 0.37 percent according to Lauret. The Commandant of Chad was pleased with Lauret's report because it had taken into consideration the epidemic that swept Melfi in 1936, killing at least 90 of the 155 who had died during that period.[65]

Although one of the objectives of this discussion is to present a partial demographic picture of the Sara and to give a general idea of the demographic situation in other parts of Chad, there are no figures specifically for the Sara that compare birth rates with mortality rates. There are, however, some fertility and mortality statistics relating to other ethnic groups, as demonstrated in Table 4 which outlines the conditions in two districts. A similar phenomenon is present in both districts; in some years mortality rates were higher than the birth rates. Did venereal diseases reduce the birth rate? Retel-Laurentin does not categorically say that venereal diseases cause sterility or infertility. Reyna expresses this uncertainty of the situation in a study of the Barma of Chad when he concludes that "our inference is just that—an inference. There is no evidence that the women classified as sterile in the population surveyed were actually sterile because of venereal infections."[66]

Recent studies, however, are less cautious and state that indeed venereal diseases, particularly gonorrhea, can cause sterility. This happens when the "infection spreads from the lower genital tract to the Fallopian tubes"; the chances of infection, however, occur "in less than one half of those women exposed to the organism." Pregnant women seem to be almost immune to the infection; it normally strikes nonpregnant women, especially those in the "lower socioeconomic status." While on the one hand gonorrhea

Table 4. *Birth and Death Rates in Two Chari-Baguirmi Districts*

Year	Massenya		Goz-Boda	
	Births	*Deaths*	*Births*	*Deaths*
1930	—	—	1.6%	4.0%
1931	2.8%	2.7%	1.2	2.0
1932	2.7	2.5	1.8	7.0
1933	2.0	1.0	2.7	1.1
1934	2.9	1.0	2.0	1.0
1935	3.1	1.8	2.3	1.2
1936	2.9	1.6	1.8	4.0
1937	3.0	2.5	1.4	1.5
1938	2.7	2.6	1.9	7.0
1939	3.0	1.0	2.1	7.7
1940	3.0	1.8	2.2	7.0
1941	2.9	1.8	2.7	7.7
1942	3.1	1.9	2.0	1.1

Source: W83, 3, 1951, p. 14.

seems to have a link (not yet completely understood) with the so-called pelvic inflammatory disease (PID), causing sterility or "ectopic pregnancy" in about 15 percent of the patients. Syphilis, on the other hand, induces "miscarriages, stillbirths, or children with pre-natal syphilis" in women infected immediately prior to pregnancy.[67] Thus it is difficult to avoid the impression that venereal diseases in Chad had a negative impact on demographic conditions in Sara districts as well as in the other sections of the country during and after the colonial period.

Influenza

The influenza pandemic of 1918–19 is much easier to assess because it had a devastating impact on Chad. "If the German epidemic had lasted a month, all Sara would have perished." This is the typical statement one hears from Sara elders. They call it a German epidemic because they believe that the "influenza" was caused by gas spread over Chad and Cameroon at the end of World War I. In their opinion, the Germans used gas after realizing that the French were defeating them in battle. In the Sara language, the name for that particular epidemic is *ngalbogui.* That its name is still remembered, although it struck over half a century ago, attests to the impact it had.

Spanish influenza, as it is generally known, hit Europe first and later swept over the continent of Africa. Its death toll has been calculated at twenty million worldwide. I. R. Phimister describes it as the worst pandemic in the history of man on earth. "With the exceptions of New Guinea, St. Helena and certain South Pacific Islands, the whole world was ultimately ravaged by the disease, which attacked 50 percent of the world's population, the attendant death rate averaging 3 percent."[68]

Influenza apparently reached the West African coast by sea in August and September 1918, then moved southward to Zaire, and in the following months mercilessly spread through central Africa. Despite some frontier precautions taken by health officials and administrators in Chad, the pandemic swept into the territory from Dahomey (Benin), Nigeria, and Cameroon. It emerged in the capital, Fort-Lamy, on December 14, 1918, and lasted until the end of July 1919. It claimed the largest number of victims in Moyen-Chari in January of 1919. The symptoms, as Grosfillez, an army doctor in Chad, described them, were: infection of practically all the internal organs, including the respiratory; mucus expectoration and tremors; fevers, heat waves, high body temperatures, insomnia and constipation; and pulmonary and cardiac complications which could cause death. The attack lasted from two to ten days.[69] Treatment consisted mainly of the administration of quinine, purgative washing, and camphor oil injections.

In Koumra subprefecture, the epidemic lasted only six days.[70] The people of Bessada report that it killed at least one out of five inhabitants in eight days. At Bouna the disease lasted only a few days and killed dozens of people, especially children.[71] At Bedaya, less than 50 kilometers from Koumra town, the disease likewise lasted only a week, but is said to have killed 25 out of 80 people or about 31 percent. At Bekamba, after seven days of tribulation, the villagers buried 40 people in a span of three days. The present Chef de Poste Administratif of this region was fourteen years old when the epidemic occurred. He recalled that after one person was buried, the grave diggers, ready to return to the village, received orders to remain and dig more and more graves. At Ndila it was the same story: five out of fifteen people died. At the village of Peni, an old man remembered the sudden and inexplicable death of 30 people in the next village *carré* or *quartier*. In his own *carré*, of the 80 inhabitants, 20 died that week. Bekonjo village lost 45 people in a week.

Occasionally villagers took extraordinary measures to "stop" the ravages of the influenza. At Kol, for instance, after the failure of local chefs de terre, a marabout or Muslim teacher was called to the village to use whatever powers he had to stop the disease. The marabout circled the village three times, performing special atonement rituals. The effect of the epidemic was thereafter curtailed with fewer deaths subsequently reported.[72] Fortunately for the marabout, he was invited after the initial devastation was over. At Beko, the consequences were practically the same. In the village of Dokobo, near Doba, the death toll reportedly claimed 60 percent of the community. At Doyaba, the epidemic lasted over a week. In 1974 the oldest living resident recalled the death of ten persons near the compound of his father, the village chief.[73] In 90 percent of the villages visited, the elders assumed that the epidemic was introduced by people, especially school children who had gone to Sarh (Fort-Archambault) to participate in a French national holiday. Some of them returned to the village to die near their parents; others succumbed in Sarh itself or on their way back to the villages.

The archival material is once more sketchy on statistics although the disturbing sweep of influenza is mentioned several times. Georges Bruel talks of the "grands ravages" of the "grippe espagnole" in 1918 in Equatorial Africa.[74] One can assume that deaths were higher than the 15,483 officially reported for Moyen-Chari, a figure which represented about 8 percent of the district's population. Oral information suggests that death claimed one-third of the population in affected communities. Mortality, however, was sometimes exaggerated. Bouffard, an army doctor, cites reports estimating a death rate of 80 percent among persons who contracted the disease.[75] The doctor tells about his experience in former Dahomey with Chadian troops.

> I witnessed the epidemic of 1918 in French West Africa (Dahomey) . . . A detachment of six hundred troops from Chad arrived at Porto-Novo after crossing Nigeria. It was attacked by the epidemic three days before its arrival. The next morning, 400 out of the 600 troops had a temperature of 38° to 40°C from fever. But the epidemic caused only 34 deaths [about 6 percent of the total contingent]. Europeans were more severely hit.[76]

What was its toll in Chad? If doctors' reports are reasonably accurate, of approximately 1,075,000 Chadians, some 70,000 cases were actually reported.[77] The extent of unreported cases is problematical. Existing statistical data are inadequate to determine how many of the reported cases died, but oral sources put the number of deaths at one-third of the stricken; that is, around 23,000. Table 5 is illustrative of the problem. In Fort-Lamy and

Table 5. Influenza in Fort-Lamy and Vicinity

Number of sick	Percentage of sick	Number of deaths	Percentage of deaths	Areas infected
50 Europeans	78	7	14	Fort-Lamy, Fort-Archambault and vicinity
650 soldiers (Africans)	80	107	16	Fort-Lamy, vicinity, a few towns
30,630 Africans	78	650	2.1	Fort-Lamy and vicinity
Hundreds			Less than 1	Abeche
		1		Salamat

Source: Grosfillez, "L'épidémie d'influenza de 1918–1919," p. 457.

vicinity, for example, thousands of Africans fell victims, but only 2.1 percent were reported dead from the epidemic.

Conclusion

Some of the diseases discussed above, sleeping sickness, venereal diseases, and Spanish influenza, entered Chad from West Africa during the past hundred years. Others, like smallpox and meningitis, may have been endemic in parts of Chad; but there is a consensus that Europeans, and possibly the earlier trading caravans enabled some diseases to become epidemic. Europeans —the French in the case of Chad—obviously did not intend for this to happen. But the fact remains that, had they been genuinely concerned with the welfare of the people within the colony, they would have expanded health facilities at about the same pace as the growth of economic activities within the country. Yet only four medical centers existed from 1929 to 1945 in all of Chad. The archival material does not allow one to determine even approximate death tolls from epidemics in any given district of Chad. But the scattered evidence reveals that the epidemics were highly devastating in specific localities.

A brief review of the above information reveals a significant loss of life from epidemic diseases. Sleeping sickness occurred in Chad, particularly in the areas of Moyen-Chari, the two Logones, and part of Chari-Baguirmi, almost every year after 1906 until 1940. Some medical accounts and eyewitness reports indicate that in the prefectures of Moyen-Chari and Moyen Logone at least one-third of the population was infected by the epidemic and that about one-third of the victims died. Archival data shows that the population of the two prefectures oscillated between 300,000 and 400,000 during the period 1920–25. If these accounts are approximately correct, the death rate would have been in the neighborhood of 11 percent per year. Such a percentage, however, seems too high since preventive services had been introduced by then. But half of that figure could well reflect the impact of the disease; such a percentage is still a very high demographic price to pay.

Meningitis epidemics competed with trypanosomiasis for victims. From 1928 to 1938 reported deaths reached 10,000; considering, however, that most cases were not reported, and basing our estimates on Dr. Ledentu's study, we calculate that over 12,000 people died in a period of ten years, about 1.2 percent of the Chadian population. In Doba alone some 3 percent of the inhabitants were buried in 1938. Compared with sleeping sickness, the gravity of meningitis lies in the fact that it affected all prefectures of Chad and continues to do so at present.

Smallpox epidemics also claimed thousands of victims, as in 1925. In that year alone 3.3 percent of the prefecture of Moyen-Chari died of smallpox. In some localities the epidemic was so severe that commercial activities ceased and frontiers with neighboring countries closed. Venereal diseases also appear to have been widespread in Chad, especially in the north. Contemporary medical reports describe a disturbing spread in the south as well. Under ordinary conditions syphilis and gonorrhea do not kill their victims, but their apparent link to female infertility suggests that they had a significant demographic impact. That the central and northern populations of Chad showed a low birth rate in the past and continue to do so now may be indicative of the impact of venereal diseases. Their effects are more difficult to measure in the south.

The Spanish influenza was present in Chad for only a few months, but its impact was serious. Contemporary reports indicate that some 23,000 Chadians died from influenza in 1918–19. We know that some 15,000 people of Moyen-Chari died in the period 1918–19, about 9 percent of that prefecture. Mortality was not the same everywhere in Chad. Climate conditions, the degree of mobility, population density, health care facilities, and other factors must be taken into consideration.

Combined, the epidemics discussed here may have cost Chad over 4 percent of its population yearly, excluding deaths caused by endemic diseases and natural phenomena. The evidence suggests that the south was hardest hit, especially the Moyen-Chari region. Another result of these epidemics, of course, was continuous displacement of people and severe demographic instability. In several cases the authorities forced people to abandon their villages and settle in safer places or undergo treatment in the few centers created for such purposes, as was the case of Mousnini and Beraba.

The advent of colonialism was instrumental in spreading diseases in Chad, and the human cost of these epidemics should not be underestimated. Confronted with such a phenomenon, the outside world must attempt to understand the physical and psychological costs required of the Chadians. Their resistance and persistence confound the imagination. In Chad colonialism increased the extent and intensity of contact between geographically separated people. The program to establish large village settlements, the increased use of rivers, the government's developmental projects that brought together thousands of Africans belonging to different ethnic groups from different environments, and the use of roads unintentionally created an environment more favorable for the spread of epidemics. Of course, the French were not solely responsible for this phenomenon in Africa; the British, Germans, Portuguese, Belgians, and Italians inadvertently contributed to higher mortality in the continent. In the Belgian Congo early in this century, e.g., colonial policies had very similar results in the northeastern Semliki valley. Charles Good has observed that

the new settlements were unwittingly established in Semliki's endemic focus of sleeping sickness in proximity to permanent streams, all of which were (and are) infested with *G. palpalis,* the vector of *T. gambiense.* In consequence, the large population movements generated by the settlement process and the siting of the new villages fostered so much additional man-tsetse contact that the pre-existing endemic was quickly converted into a rampant epidemic.[78]

Good's remark is true for sleeping sickness as well as for other types of infectious diseases. The entrenchment of colonial rule simply increased mortality from epidemic diseases, as is clearly exemplified in Chad. Increased mortality in turn caused significant demographic instability and frequent depopulation. What effect this had on the attitude and values of people has yet to be determined.

Of course, the degree of credibility of the diagnosis performed by doctors over three decades ago in Africa is problematic, given that even today the nature and the symptoms of some of the infectious diseases mentioned in this study are not clearly understood. One of the simplest diseases to diagnose, for example, is smallpox, caused by poxvirus *variola*. But its diagnosis can become difficult after complications resulting in encephalitis, psychoses, and edema.[79]

Meningitis, "an inflammation of the meninges or coverings of the brain," can be caused by different agents. Wehrle distinguishes ten types, namely, bacterial, viral, tuberculous, amebic, brain abcess, coccidioidomycosis, cysticerosis, leptospirosis, toxoplasmosis, and trichinosis; the problem is even more complicated as patients with encephalitis often show "all of the clinical manifestations and cerebrospinal fluid abnormalities" of viral meningitis.[80] Did colonial doctors make a distinction, for instance, between viral and bacterial meningitis? The question is unanswerable since diagnostic and pathogenic information is missing in the documents.

Likewise, there are different types of trypanosomiasis. Doctors who failed to differentiate *T. gambiense* from *T. rhodesiense* very likely administered the wrong drug. Suramin (particularly moranyl), extensively used in Chad, is much more effective when prescribed against *T. rhodesiense*. Similar general remarks could be made of venereal diseases and influenza. The medical shortcomings of decades ago, however, do not obscure the reality of the frequent occurrences of epidemics that wiped out entire villages in the former French colony.

French authorities claim, as it were, that they used all means at their disposal to eradicate these diseases in Chad and to minimize their serious demographic impact. Their overall performance does not, unfortunately, appear impressive, as Table 6 reveals. The areas of health care that improved between 1929 and 1946 were the number of nurses, of consultations, and of vaccinations. The number of doctors and hospitals remained almost static in

Table 6. Medical Facilities in Chad, 1929–46

Items	1929	1933	1940	1946
Doctors	4	6	21	19
Auxiliary doctors	1	none	none	2
Pharmacists	none	none	1	1
Hygienists	2	3	none	none
Administrative officers	none	none	none	1
Underofficers (S.I.C.)	4	7	16	12
Sanitary agents	none	none	2	5
Midwives	7	none	7	5
African doctors	none	none	none	3
Nurses	46	123	none?	221
Number of consultations	91,631	212,505	820,852	900,000
Hospitalization of Africans	unknown	unknown	8,961	8,836
Vaccinations/ smallpox	85,335	135,000	223,945	471,276
Vaccinations/ meningitis	unknown	unknown	94,858	107,605
Leper colonies	none	none	6	306 beds
Hospitals	unknown	1 (40 beds)	1 (60 beds)	1 (80 beds)
Temporary medical establishments	3	2 (70 beds)	2 (170 beds)	2 (178 beds)
Medical centers	4	4	12 (537 beds)	8 (312 beds)
Infirmaries	none	2 (70 beds)	11 (91 beds)	17 (334 beds)

Source: W53, 18, 1946, pp. 6–7.

proportion to the population. The increase in vaccinations, how-ever, corresponds to an increase in mobile units, especially in the fight against sleeping sickness, smallpox, and meningitis. Dr. Jamot had introduced vaccination mobile units in Equatorial Africa as early as 1916, but it is apparent that doctors avoided working in French Equatorial Africa when possible. They nor-mally preferred the Belgian Congo where the pay was higher.

It is also worth noting that a great number of the doctors in Chad were trained for and attached to the army. Thus, their responsibility was the health of military personnel and not that of civilians. This means that few doctors had time to treat the victims of the epidemics; they were as mobile as the army, and their care of civilians was typically on an emergency basis only. From 1933 to 1946 there was but one hospital in the entire colony of Chad. Health records, for example, show that in 1940 about 9,000 people were hospitalized, almost at the rate of 25 patients a day. Where and how these patients were handled is an open question.

In addition, there are no convincing records in Chad suggest-ing that measures were taken to provide medical care for new settlements or for laborers recruited to work on projects associ-ated with private enterprise or government. Sara elders reported that employers forced even the sick to work since they were not sure when their employees told the truth or lied.[81] Campaigns to encourage improved hygiene and cleanliness in addition to in-structions on avoiding epidemics do not appear in the official Chadian records.

Such remarks are not intended to deny credit to whatever was done in the health sector by the French authorities or to ignore that contemporary diagnostic and therapeutic methods needed much improvement. French doctors and nurses in Chad must, in fact, be commended for their service. It took a philanthropist's courage and dedication to work in a hostile environment and in a landlocked territory such as Chad which had no railroad. Be-cause of the poor transportation and communication network, medical supplies most often had to be brought in from the coast hundreds of miles away on porters' shoulders. We must assume that doctors as a whole did their best to prevent and to eradicate epidemics. But they were too few in number for their effort to be meaningful in a colony plagued by disease. The responsibility to provide more doctors, nurses, and medical supplies, and to expand health facilities, fell on the government. Ironically, while the doctors were busy fighting the severe infectious diseases, the government was indirectly undoing their work with its projects and forced labor concentrations which became centers of disease dissemination.

High annual death rates should have compelled officials to take greater steps to minimize the effect of epidemics and to enact stronger measures to protect the inhabitants, especially the workers, from possible contagion. If this was done, the records are uncomfortably silent. The losers in this whole process were, of course, the Chadians, and especially the Sara whose services the French demanded for the labor force and as recruits for the colonial army.

Notes

1. See Henry Dobyns, "Estimating Aboriginal American Population," *Current Anthropology*, I (October 1966), 410 ff.; and Woodrow Borah and Shelburne F. Cook, *The Indian Population of Central Mexico, 1531–1610* (Berkeley, 1960).

2. B. Pentony, "Psychological Causes of Depopulation of Primitive Groups," *Oceania*, XXIV (December 1953), 142–45; Nancy Bowers, "Demographic Problems in Montane New Guinea," *Culture and Population: A Collection of Current Studies*, IX (1971), 12–16; also see G. Pitt-Rivers, *The Clash of Culture and the Contact of Races* (London, 1927).

3. William Petersen, *Population* (London, 1970), p. 355.

4. Philip Curtin, "Epidemiology and the Slave Trade," *Political Science Quarterly* LXXXIII (June 1968), 195.

5. Chadian archives are kept in numbered wooden boxes in N'Djamena (former Fort-Lamy). Each box contains several files identified by the letter W, a number attached to it, a second number in most cases, and the year to which the material refers. Pages are often not numbered. The footnoting will reflect this order; example: W19, 5, 1920, p. 5.
Oral data was collected through interviews of over 200 Sara elders, forty years old and over, representing approximately 25 Sara villages and towns.

6. K. R. S. Morris, "The Spread of Sleeping Sickness Across Central Africa," *Journal of Tropical Medicine and Hygiene*, LXVI (March 1963), 60.

7. John J. McKelvey, Jr., *Man Against Tsetse; Struggle for Africa* (Ithaca, 1973), p. 3.

8. Albert Schweitzer, *A l'orée de la forêt vierge* (Paris, 1952), pp. 105–7.

9. McKelvey, *Man Against Tsetse*, p. 5.

10. R. Hoeppli, *Parasitic Diseases in Africa and the Western Hemisphere* (Basel, 1969), p. 215. Hoeppli suggests that the slave trade transmitted the disease to the West Indies and South Africa, pp. 31–34.

11. Morris, "Spread of Sleeping Sickness," p. 76.

12. Anne Retel-Laurentin, *Infécondité en Afrique noire* (Paris, 1974), pp. 42–43.

13. Morris, "Spread of Sleeping Sickness," p. 77.

14. Alfred Buck *et al.*, *Health and Disease in Chad* (Baltimore, 1970), pp. 84, 136.

15. For a brief analysis of the epidemic in former French Equatorial Africa see Retel-Laurentin, *Infécondité en Afrique noire*, pp. 44–47.

16. R. Kuczynski, *The Cameroons and Togoland* (London, 1939), p. 183. Réné-Jules Cornet in *Medicine et exploration—contacts de quelques explorateurs de l'Afrique centrale avec les maladies tropicales* (Brussels, 1970), p. 77, indicates that one indigenous authority in Central Africa had presumably initiated a forest clean-up program to fight the disease.

17. Bertin Moyangar, "Le rôle des missions catholiques dans l'histoire du Tchad de 1900 à 1970" (unpublished M.A. thesis, Université de Lyon, 1972), p. 92.

18. Father Clovis of Doba supported this version and based his opinion on a similar practice of French missionaries in Indochina.

19. Alcantara, "La maladie du sommeil," *Le Courier du Logone—Nouvelles du Diocèse de Moundou. Tchad*, XLIV (April 1969), 10.

20. Alcantara, LII (1971), 10; see also XLVI (1971), 10.

21. Interview with Bamaloum of Mousnini, Moissala, 26 June 1974. When I asked the people of Moissala to direct me to Mousnini, they turned their backs and said, "You are wasting your time; because of the sad origin of their village, the people of Mousnini will never open their mouths to you." Disregarding their advice, I crossed the Barh Sara River and was cordially received by Mousnini villagers. Bamaloum and his friends were more than willing to tell the tragic story of the village.

22. The elders are still convinced that the cause of the epidemic was an unusual yam, harvested in 1923, which was too large and too juicy. People who ate it supposedly died. Flies bit the infested yam and transmitted the disease to distant villages. It is impossible, of course, that the yam was the cause. But at least the vector—the fly—is part of the story.

23. Interview with Father Réné, Catholic Mission of Bodo, Doba, 22 July 1974.

24. Interview with Guirdi, village chief, and his team, Beraba, Doba, 21 July 1974.

25. D. Scott, "The Epidemic of Gambian Sleeping Sickness," in H. W. Mulligan (ed.), *African Trypanosomiasis* (New York, 1970), p. 640.

26. Retel-Laurentin, *Infécondité en Afrique noire*, pp. 46–47.

27. Frank Hawking, "African Trypanosomiasis," George Hunter, J. Clyde Swartzwelder, and David F. Clyde (eds.), *Tropical Medicine* (Philadelphia, 1976), p. 437. The problem of tryparsamide is illustrated by an episode involving one of Dr. Jamot's students. Jamot received 250 grams of tryparsamide from the Rockefeller Institute in 1923. One of his aides in the Cameroons overdosed his patients, and seven hundred of them went blind. The incident created such an uproar that the aide was expelled from the colony. Dr. Jamot, who had advised his aide never to exceed the prescribed dosage, nevertheless defended him. Because of this stand, Jamot was later arrested in Dakar. His career was damaged

by this series of events and the campaign against sleeping sickness, which Jamot directed, was impaired; see McKelvey, *Man Against Tsetse*, pp. 130–31.

28. Alcantara, "La maladie du sommeil," LII (1971), 11 ff., and Hawking, "African Trypanosomiasis," p. 434.

29. Morris, "Spread of Sleeping Sickness," p. 5.

30. Retel-Laurentin, *Infécondité en Afrique noire*, p. 43.

31. McKelvey, *Man Against Tsetse*, p. 58.

32. Retel-Laurentin, *Infécondité en Afrique noire*, p. 46.

33. Charles Wilcocks and P. E. C. Manson-Bahr (eds.), *Manson's Tropical Diseases* (Baltimore, 1972 edition), p. 554.

34. *Ibid.*

35. B. B. Waddy, "African Epidemic Cerebro-Spinal Meningitis," *Journal of Tropical Medicine and Hygiene*, LX (September 1957), 218–19.

36. *Ibid.*, p. 218; see also Part I of the same article, pp. 179–89.

37. The following documents give further evidence of the presence of the epidemic prior to 1938: W32, (n.n.), 1920, p. 2; W37, 43, 1920, p. 45; W37, 5, 1924, p. 3; W37, (n.n), 1925, p. 15; W29, 3, 1937, (n.p.).

38. W29, 6, 1938, p. 25.

39. Col. Ledentu, "La méningite cérébro-spinale en Afrique équatoriale française pendant le premier semestre 1938," *Bulletin mensuel de l'office internationale d'hygiène publique*, XXX (1939), 1–5.

40. W29, 6, 1938, p. 25.

41. Ledentu, "La méningite cérébro-spinale en Afrique," p. 443.

42. W29, 6, 1938, p. 49.

43. W38, 3, 1951, pp. 1–7.

44. W36, 45, 1922, (n.p.). In 1920 at least 110 people died in Massacory from smallpox; see W19, 2, 1920, p. 14.

45. W32, 38–40, 1929, (n.p).

46. W19, 10, 1932, pp. 45–46.

47. Saul Krugman, Robert Ward, and Samuel Katz, *Infectious Diseases in Children* (St. Louis, 1977), p. 313.

48. Stephen Reyna, "The Costs of Marriage: A Study of some Factors Affecting Barma Fertility" (unpublished Ph.D. dissertation, Columbia University, 1974), p. 129.

49. Retel-Laurentin, *Infécondité en Afrique noire*, p. 48.

50. See *ibid.* and Anatole Romaniuk, *La fécondité des populations congolaises* (Paris, 1967).

51. Interview with the chief of carré, Beralngar, Koumra, 21 June 1974.

52. Interview with the village chief of Kol, his *chef de terre*, and their team, Kol, Koumra, 26 July 1974.

53. Interview with Fathers Raoul, Clovis, and Paul, Doba, 18, 19, 20, and 24 July 1974.

54. Retel-Laurentin, *Infécondité en Afrique noire*, pp. 50–51.

55. E. H. Hudson, "Treponematosis and Man's Social Evolution," *American Anthropologist*, LXVII (August 1965), 885, 895.

56. For a general discussion of the controversy surrounding the origin of syphilis see Alfred W. Crosby, Jr., *The Columbian Exchange: Biological and Cultural Consequences of 1492* (Westport, Conn., 1972), pp. 122–64.

57. W36, 6, 1910, p. 5; W36, 45, 1922, p. 13; W36, 57, 1923, p. 5.

58. Georges Bruel, *L'Afrique équatoriale française* (Paris, 1919), p. 327.

59. W37, 37, 1928, p. 3.

60. See W17, 18 (*sic*); quoted in Reyna, "The Costs of Marriage," pp. 125–30.

61. Retel-Laurentin, *Infécondité en Afrique noire,* p. 63.

62. *Ibid.,* p. 66.

63. Christian Bouquet, "Les incertitudes de la démographie africaine: l'éxemple du Tchad," *Les Cahiers d'Outre-Mer, Revue de géographie,* XCVI (October/December 1971), 410.

64. W90, 11, 1936, pp. 1–19.

65. *Ibid.,* p. 19.

66. Reyna, "The Costs of Marriage," p. 277.

67. S. J. Berman and Robert W. Kistner, *Progress in Infertility* (Boston, 1975 edition), p. 208. See also Ambrose King and Claude Nicol, *Venereal Diseases* (Baltimore, 1975 edition), pp. 205–7.

68. I. R. Phimister, "The 'Spanish' Influenza Pandemic of 1918 and its Impact on the Southern Rhodesian Mining Industry," *The Central African Journal of Medicine,* XIX (July 1973), 143.

69. M. le Dr. Grosfillez, "L'épidémie d'influenza de 1918–1919," *Annales de Medicine et de Pharmacie coloniales,* XIX (1921), 457–58.

70. Interview with an *ancient combattant,* former railroad workers, a *chef de carré,* and others, Koumra, 14, 21, and 24 June 1974.

71. Interview with the Bouna village chief and his team, Bouna, Moissala, 27 June 1974.

72. Interview with the Kol village chief, *chef de terre,* and their team, Kol, Koumra, 26 July 1974.

73. Interview with a retired World War II sergeant, Doyoba, Sarh, 30 July 1974.

74. Bruel, *L'Afrique équatoriale française,* p. 170.

75. Méd. Gen. Bouffard, "La Pneumococci chez les noirs," *Bulletin de la Société des Récherches congolaises,* XVII (1932), 4.

76. *Ibid.,* p. 8.

77. Retel-Laurentin compares its effect to that of sleeping sickness, see *Infécondité en Afrique noire,* p. 44.

78. Charles Good, "Salt, Trade and Disease; Aspects of Development in Africa's Northern Great Lakes Region," *International Journal of African Historical Studies,* V (August 1972), 543–86.

79. Krugman *et al.,* p. 313.

80. Paul Wehrle, "Meningitis," in Franklin Top and Paul Wehrle (eds.), *Communicable and Infectious Diseases* (St. Louis, 1976), p. 445; and Mary Carruthers, "Viral Meningitis and Encephalitis," in Guy P. Youmans, Philip Y. Paterson, and Herbert M. Sommers (eds.), *The Biologic and Clinical Basis of Infectious Diseases* (Philadelphia, 1975), p. 566.

81. A study of the physical impact of forced labor on the Sara and the other populations of Chad should prove interesting and revealing of the nature of colonial policies. While interviewing the elders, I was struck by the number of hernia cases. Over 90 percent of them, with the exception of a few former *tirailleurs* or soldiers, had severe cases. It would be interesting to determine if there was a relationship between these cases and colonial practices.

6

Health and Disease on the Plantations of Cameroon, 1884–1939

Mark W. DeLancey

The onset of the colonial period in Africa had as one of its many effects increased interaction between Africans and Europeans. European employers needed large numbers of Africans to work on mines, plantations, and other labor-extensive projects, and the conditions under which such labor was recruited often caused large-scale population movements, movements which necessitated important environmental changes for these workers in terms of climate, food, and living conditions. In southwestern Cameroon, where the extensive development of plantations has been a major factor in economic and social change since the beginning of the German colonial regime, the recruitment of labor for these plantations has caused widespread migration since the early 1900s. This migration and the subsequent changes in environment are, according to considerable evidence, directly related to the high rates of death and disease encountered in many locations in the early years of colonization. It remains for us to demonstrate the extent to which this migration affected mortality rates, but there can be no doubt that however positively one might wish to view the role of the plantations today, they have been, especially for the first 34 years of their existence, the cause of great suffering in twentieth-century Kamerun. (Under German rule the colony was "Kamerun." In English it is "Cameroon" and in French "Cameroun.")

The German Period

The motivations behind the German occupation of Kamerun in 1884 are not clear. Harry Rudin claims that trade was the main purpose; plantation possibilities were mentioned only "as a kind of afterthought."[1] Adolf Woermann, an important supporter of German colonial expansion in Kamerun, wrote instructions to one of his agents in which plantations were mentioned as an important consideration. After directing the agent to convince the local chiefs to turn the sovereign control of their lands over to the Kaiser, Woermann continued:

At the same time as the cession of sovereignty you should by all means get the cession of very extensive lands as private property—especially those suitable for plantations. There is no doubt that, if the country becomes German, there will be many attempts to establish extensive plantations. . . .[2]

Erik Hallden, who has studied in detail the interactions of German colonial officials, planters, and Basel missionaries over the lands alienated for plantations around Mt. Cameroon, reverses Rudin's argument completely: "The idea of plantations was decisive from the very beginning of the German colonial era, as well for the Reichs-Government as for various private interests."[3] Whatever the initial thinking might have been, by the end of the German period the plantations were a major target of investment for German capitalists,[4] a major source of cash employment for the inhabitants of the territory, and a major cause of disruption for African societies and peoples. In 1913, just prior to the British conquest of the area, there were fifty-eight plantations with 17,827 African employees and 70,562 acres under cultivation.[5]

Plantations need extensive areas of land and large, inexpensive supplies of labor. The first requirement leads to development in areas of low population density, and typically means that those persons already living in the area of development must be moved to clear spaces large enough for the economical operation of the plantations. The Germans, instead of finding empty territory when they took possession of the lands around Mt. Cameroon,

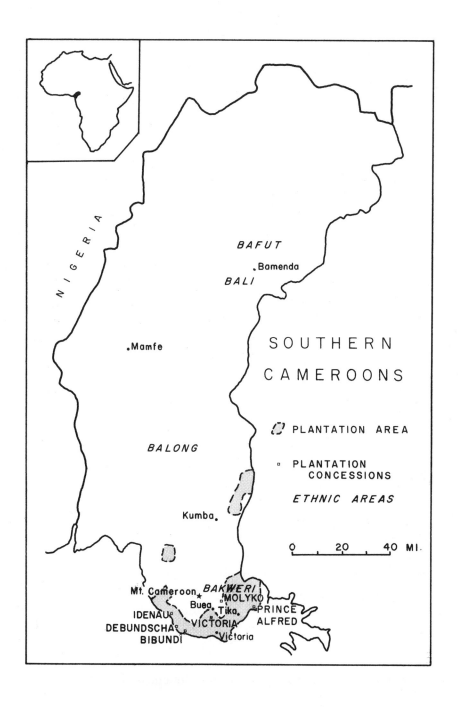

NIGERIA

BAFUT

.Bamenda

BALI

.Mamfe

SOUTHERN
CAMEROONS

PLANTATION AREA

PLANTATION
CONCESSIONS

ETHNIC AREAS

BALONG

Kumba.

0   20   40 MI.

Mt. Cameroon ★ BAKWERI
                  ▫MOLYKO
         Buea. Tiko. ▫PRINCE
IDENAU▫   ALFRED
DEBUNDSCHA VICTORIA
   BIBUNDI   .Victoria

encountered a number of scattered Bakweri villages. The Bakweri were moved from land suitable for plantations and prevented from using this land for grazing livestock and other purposes. In the process, the Germans deprived the Bakweri of their traditional homes and left them with a very small amount of land for their personal use.[6]

The second requirement for plantation development, labor, could not be solved locally because the African population of the proposed plantation district was sparse. Not only was it insufficient to fulfill labor requirements, but the local people were not particularly interested in this type of work. A few were engaged as middlemen in the trade between Africans and Europeans, although most were content to continue their normal way of life as subsistence farmers and hunters. Some employers believed that the Bakweri were simply not suitable for plantation work, and many Germans thought them inept and indolent, an opinion later shared by British officials.[7]

Initially, the required laborers were brought from outside Kamerun. The most complete information is reported by Adolf Rüger, an East German historian whose study is based on extensive archival research. The majority of workers from the time of the German annexation until 1891 were foreigners, mainly from Liberia but also from Togo, Sierra Leone, and Dahomey.[8] After this the high cost of recruiting and shipping such laborers caused employers to look elsewhere,[9] although Liberia continued to be an important source as late as 1900. Other recruiting efforts were made in Nigeria, the Congo, and Sudan, without lasting success, and the overall number of extraterritorial African laborers declined rapidly, as indicated in Table 1.

Foreign laborers declined in importance as the colonial government became capable of extracting workers from the Kamerun populations. Employees from other colonies were expensive and once administrative authority was established in Kamerun, local labor was cheaper. Moreover, administrators in other territories realized a need for labor and placed restrictions on external migration.[10]

As Kamerun's needs expanded, the difficulties in obtaining suf-

Table 1. *Foreign Workers in Total Labor Force, 1899–1902*

Date	Total laborers	Foreign laborers	Percentage Foreign labor
1 July 1899	3943	1120	28.4
1 July 1900	3850	1500	39.0
1 July 1901	3650	975	26.7
1 July 1902	2850	400	14.0

Source: Rüger, "Die Entstehung und Lage der Arbeiterklasse," p. 210.

ficient extraterritorial African workers increased, merely because the size of the undertaking was enormous; by 1913 there were almost 18,000 workers. Therefore, the German planters encouraged migration from within Kamerun, and to a large extent forced it, causing much suffering and many other problems that were made worse by competition for laborers between traders and plantation owners. The government, particularly when railroad construction began, was a third competitor for this labor, one of the Kamerun's few exploitable resources.[11]

German explorers found potential workers in the interior, where there were regions with both a sufficiently high population density and inhabitants who were accustomed to an agricultural way of life. Planters signed agreements with chiefs who could supply some of the needed workers, and persuaded the government to provide workers under regulations which we now call forced labor. Crimes were punished by sentences of labor and convicts could be turned over to private employers for a fee of 10 marks per head and 10 marks per month.[12] Peace treaties ending wars between the Germans and defeated African communities stipulated that a number of workers be supplied to work at the plantations and at other locations.[13] Near the end of the German period, limited head taxes and hut taxes strongly encouraged Africans to work in European enterprises.[14] Persons unable to pay tax in cash could be turned over to private employers, who paid the tax and the fee of 10 marks per head.[15] Heinrich Schnee, a former governor of German East Africa, dis-

puted the charges of forced labor in Kamerun, but, as discussed
below, he overlooked certain aspects of German colonial rule
and the unfortunate effects of labor migration, whether or not it
was voluntary.[16]

The centers of the internal labor supply were Bali, Fumban,
and Yaoundé, inland areas which differed in vegetation and
climate from the coastal regions where the plantations were
located. Rainfall in the plantation area is influenced by proximity to the sea and by Mt. Cameroon, a 13,350 foot volcanic
mass which rises from the coastline to its peak a few miles inland. Many of the plantations are situated by the base or at the
lower levels of the mountain. The areas on the seaward side of
the mountain receive unusually heavy amounts of rainfall;
Debundscha's average precipitation of more than 400 inches per
year makes it one of the wettest places in the world. Several
plantations were located there. The data in Table 2 indicate
some of the differences between the plantation areas and the
labor supply areas. Altitude, temperature, and rainfall all influence health, agriculture, vegetation, and way of life. The plantations were located in areas generally classified as swamp forest
or rain forest and the labor supply areas were in high savanna or
derived savanna. The coastal lowlands where the plantations

Table 2. *Selected Measures of Temperature, Rainfall, and Altitude
in Cameroon*

Location	Average annual rainfall:	Average annual temperature:	Altitude
Plantation areas:			
Debundscha	1000cm	no data	10 meters
Tiko	265cm	28°C	53 meters
Victoria	405cm	24°C	3 meters
Labor supply areas:			
Bamenda/Bali	258cm	21°C	1,524 meters
Fumban	165cm	no data	900–1500 meters
Yaoundé	158cm	no data	600–900 meters

Sources: J. A. Ngwa, *An Outline Geography of the Federal Republic of the
Cameroon* (London, 1967), pp. 28–31. Also see K. M. Buchanan and J. C. Pugh,
Land and People in Nigeria (London, 1955), pp. 1–57.

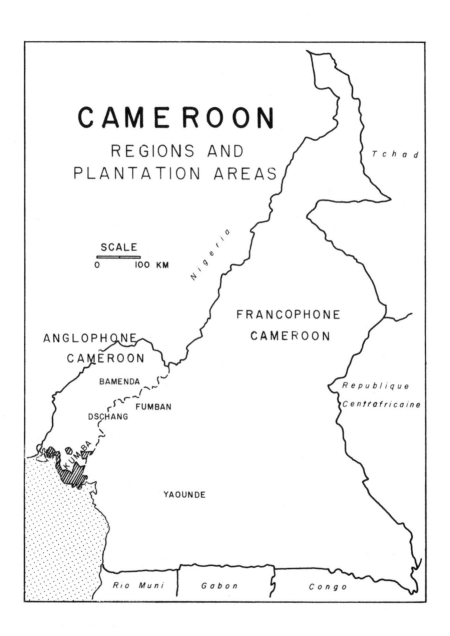

CAMEROON

REGIONS AND
PLANTATION AREAS

Tchad

SCALE
0   100 KM

Nigeria

FRANCOPHONE
CAMEROON

ANGLOPHONE
CAMEROON

BAMENDA

FUMBAN

DSCHANG

KUMBA

Republique
Centrafricaine

YAOUNDE

Rio Muni   Gabon   Congo

were located are generally hotter, wetter, and more subject to malaria and filariasis than the labor supply areas.[17] The plantation region possesses "an ideal balance of optimum conditions . . . for the propagation of the most malignant species of malaria parasite."[18] In 1949 medical surveys were conducted in Bafut, a grassland area, and in two locations in the forest plantation area, eastern Balong and northwestern Kumba. Of the 8,264 grassland dwellers surveyed in Bafut, 5.53 percent had malaria and 9.08 percent suffered from filariasis. In the sample of 8,008 forest residents, 39.16 percent had malaria and 50.64 percent had filarial infections.[19]

To the traumatic effects of moving men from one geographical area to another must be added the effects of the long and debilitating march to the coast, the crowded conditions in the barracks and camps where the laborers lived, the lack of knowledge and training of the workers concerning hygiene in such an unaccustomed social situation, unfamiliar food, and the general inadequacy of medical care provided by the plantation companies, particularly in the early years. The men were massed in large groups in the supply areas and then marched to the plantations, a trek which often took 12 days or longer. Provisions were gathered along the way, purchased or stolen from villages on the route. During the journey there was no protection from the burning sun or from the frequent rains. Once at the plantations, the men lived in large barracks—long sheds with cement or packed-dirt floors, and corrugated iron walls and roofs. Most of these measured 80 by 20 feet and were 12 feet high at the apex of the roof. Up to one hundred men might be lodged in one such building.[20] These conditions were highly conducive to the spread of communicable diseases, yet official German reports indicate that until November 1905 not a single plantation had a physician.[21]

In their essay, "Disease and 'Development' in Africa," Charles Hughes and John Hunter list six changes occurring with "development" that influence health. Three of these changes are important here: (1) overall changes in man-habitat relationships; (2) increased population movements, mixing and concentration;

and (3) changes in microenvironmental conditions (e.g., changes in housing, neighborhood, and settlement patterns).[22] In Kamerun hundreds of persons were moved from one climatic-vegetational environment to another, and laborers from various regions were mixed and concentrated in unhealthy labor camps. It is not surprising that reports of high disease and death rates on the plantations were common during this period.

For the most part, this analysis has relied on secondary sources for information on morbidity and mortality among plantation workers during the German period. These sources include the works of historians such as Rudin and the demographer, Robert Kuczynski. In addition, official German correspondence and reports were often quoted by British officers after the conquest of Kamerun. These materials, now located in the Buea Branch of the Cameroon National Archives, contain many references to the labor problems of the German administration. All this evidence indicates that disease was widespread and that a large proportion of the workers died as a result of the migration experience.

Kuczynski quotes several medical officers stationed in the colony, but for only one year (1905–6) was there an estimated mortality rate among plantation laborers: of 5,910 laborers, 625 died, a death rate of more than 100 per thousand. The death rates at Victoria Plantation ranged from 33.1 to 102.4 per thousand during the period 1909 to 1913, and the overall rate for these years was 79.8 per thousand. For the Prince Albrecht Plantation the death rates were 137 per thousand in 1911, 268 per thousand in 1912, and 79.6 per thousand in 1913.[23] Of 1,430 persons sent on forced labor from Bamenda District in 1913 to work on three coastal plantations, 157 died in nine months, an annual rate of 146 per thousand.[24]

Several problems are associated with the use of these crude death rates. We have no description, for example, of the population involved. We know that it was largely, perhaps totally, male, and we suspect that it probably consisted of young men and boys. Rudin, however, notes that chiefs used their position in the recruiting system to deport political enemies, likely to be older men, and that "they sometimes sent away the weakest and least desirable members of the tribe."[25] If such practices were widespread, then high death rates are less surprising. Another problem, however, relates to the number of deaths reported by the plantations. The figures might actually be low, as workers were often sent home at the first sign of illness, and the plantation reports do not indicate deaths while en route to or from plantations. We lack data with which to compare these death rates. What was the crude death rate of the Kamerun population or of the male population for these years? Death rates for preindustrial tropical populations probably were about 40 per thousand.[26] Most of the figures quoted in the available materials are far above 40 per thousand; we can conclude that the death rate on the plantations was unusually high. The common causes of death are listed as dysentery, tuberculosis, typhus, pneumonia, and "poisoning." Inadequate food, poor water supplies, and helminthic infections are mentioned as contributing factors.

Opinions of German observers and the reaction of the population to the plantation labor experience suggest widespread recognition that the plantation death rate was disturbing and unusual. Lieutenant von Adametz, a German station commander at Bamenda, reported that in 1912 there were 94 deaths in a Bali work gang of 300 men at the plantations. He claimed that "the Bali population, as a result of this 'mass-recruiting', is being reduced. The flower of the Bali nation lies on the Cameroon Mountain."[27] Mansfeld, the officer in charge of Ossidinge District, reported in 1913 that "there can be no further question of recruiting voluntary labourers. . . . Only by executive measures, such as the punishment of the chiefs, threats of burning down villages, and forcible despatching under military escorts, can one attain the result of obtaining from 1,500 to 1,800 men to go to the coast, and, moreover to labour centres which are universally hated."[28] The report for Johann Albrechtshohe District for that year complained that the high number of adult males absent for labor elsewhere (8,943 men) was damaging to the local economy. "The district will be, by degrees, completely ruined unless the demands for the supply of labour are considerably reduced. . . ."[29] The entire population of several villages fled to Nigeria because of the labor demands made upon them.

In 1918, after the British conquest, district officers were requested to determine the preference of their constituents for British or German rule. The results of such an exercise must be taken skeptically because of the bias of the officer collecting the information and the fear of the person giving his opinion. Nevertheless, the vehemence of opinions expressed on the forced labor system is striking. Of 34 Ossidinge chiefs who gave statements, 26 mentioned the plantation labor situation as a cause of their discontent. Most of these mentioned the high death rate and the numerous floggings which took place on the estates.[30] Bali was a major source of labor and their ruler, the Fon, was one of the major recipients of income from that labor. However, a British colonial official reported a significant conversation with the Fon of Bali some years after the British take-over. The Fon compared the British unfavorably to the Germans in terms of road building, expansion of trade, and control over missionaries, "but he did at least concede that he was glad that the old days of forced labour on the German plantations was a thing of the past."[31]

Heinrich Schnee, in his defense of German colonial rule, argued that the accusation of German plantation labor as the cause of depopulation was merely propaganda:

The apparent depopulation of certain districts in the Cameroons was due, not to work on the plantations, but to another cause altogether. . . . The actual cause was the exploitation of the wild rubber trees growing in one part of the colony. This exploitation led to undue demands being made upon the natives living on or near the caravan routes affected. These men were required as carriers and also to attend to the needs of passing caravans. . . . The result was that the natives sought to avoid the constant disturbances and the work . . . by moving away from the neighborhood. These then tended to become deserts, not on account of the population dying off, but on account of it moving away.[32]

His arguments are not convincing, even for the last years of German control. The death rate was high among workers at the plantations. German administrators issued laws and the planters responded only as the need for more workers became critical.

British officials who studied these laws were impressed by the provisions for the workers' health.[33] But as the death rates quoted above indicate, the legislation had little effect, and German officials in the Kamerun admitted that the losses at the plantations were being felt in the supplying villages and towns.

Thus, for the people of Cameroon the German period was a time of brutal experiences as laborers on the plantations. Large numbers of Africans were migrating from their homelands to areas with critically different disease environments. Many of them never returned.

The Postwar Years

With the defeat of Germany in World War I and the division among the victors of her colonial possessions as League of Nations mandates, Kamerun became, in the west, the British mandate of the Cameroons, and, in the east, the French mandate of Cameroun. The plantations, most of which were located in the British sector, were placed under government control, but after an unsuccessful attempt to auction these properties to nonenemy nationals in 1922, most of the estates returned to their German owners at a second auction in 1924. German ownership lasted until 1939 when the plantations were taken over by the British and have remained under government control since that time.

From the very beginning of British rule the administration clearly stated its desire to avoid the forced labor system of the Germans. The British, however, also wished to maintain those aspects of the economy which had been developed during the German period. For the Cameroon populations, these conflicting policies meant a temporary continuation of the misery of forced labor.

Upon conquering the area the British were immediately faced with a shortage of workers, for many laborers had run off during the fighting.[34] This problem was partially solved by the use of a large number of refugees as laborers in return for shelter, food, and pay. But more workers were needed and instructions were sent to political officers to supply voluntary recruits. In May 1916 the Resident in Buea instructed the District Officer in Ossidinge Division to undertake *"voluntary recruiting"* [District Officer's emphasis] to supply two thousand workers needed immediately. "It should be thoroughly understood that this recruiting must consist of purely voluntary labour, and that no pressure of any sort must be applied."[35] From Lagos a year later Governor Sir Frederick Lugard wrote: "There must be no forced or 'semi-forced' labour whatever, unless on terms and conditions definitely approved in writing by me."[36]

For the general public, and for some of the political officers, the new system was difficult to distinguish from that existing during the German period. In most instances the orders were sent from Buea to district officers in the field, who passed on instructions to chiefs. Chiefs, in turn, apparently resorted to some forms of pressure to get the needed volunteers. Thus the District Officer for Bamenda, G. S. Podevin, noted that of 1,100 recruits sent in by chiefs in 1918, he had to return 400 to their villages because they claimed they had been forced to volunteer.[37]

Several officials admitted that they had threatened chiefs and had actually used force to get volunteers. The District Officer of Victoria Division sent a message to chiefs in June 1917 notifying them that they were to assist a plantation recruiter who would soon visit their villages. Chiefs were to "persuade" the people to work. "I expect all Chiefs to assist, and should they fail to do so and a large number of men not come forward, I shall send for them [the chiefs] to come to Buea and explain why they failed to carry out my orders."[38] Letters from district officers mentioned that they were having difficulty getting volunteers and suggested that compulsion might be needed. At least one official, J. Rutherfoord, Assistant District Officer, Kumba, admitted that direct pressure had been used: "I would emphasize that all labour sent by me has been compulsorily recruited. In two or three instances a policeman has had to be sent after messengers who have failed to secure the labourers. I have had to fine and imprison persons who have deserted or who have refused to go when ordered."[39] The Resident admitted in 1916 that workers had been recruited in a drastic manner "and could in no sense be regarded as free labour. . . . It was impossible to attract free labour from the surrounding districts, unless the conditions were improved."[40] Such conditions included better pay and food rations, and the guaranteed promise of management to comply with the contracts it made with workers.

The labor shortages which had harassed plantation managers in previous years continued in 1918. In August 1917 the Resident's Office in Buea instructed district officers to send 7,800 recruits to begin work in January 1918. These men were to come on contracts ranging from three to six months. The first of these contracts ended in March, and on 1 April 1918 new orders were issued from Buea to recruit several thousand more workers. The officials in the field apparently were not able to fill these quotas, but large numbers of men and boys were sent to work. The Bamenda region had supplied 1,700 recruits by the end of January and a further 455 were sent in May. The District Officer of Chang reported that 1,879 recruits had been sent from his area in 1918.[41] No information has been located to indicate the exact total of recruits from other divisions, but large numbers of laborers were sent from these areas.[42]

In March and April the first of these workers returned home and numerous complaints about conditions at the plantations were reported by the district officers. These complaints referred to late payment or nonpayment of wages, the failure of plantations to provide promised rations, the failure to provide rations while trekking between home and plantation, and a high death rate among the recruits from the grassland regions of Bamenda and Chang.[43]

For the health of Cameroonians in general and for plantation workers in particular, 1918 was a disastrous year. Extremely high death rates at the plantations meant that this was to be the last year of political recruiting. The influenza pandemic which swept the world reached British Cameroons in November. The Resident estimated that 35,000 persons out of a total population of 153,360 died; that is, almost 23 percent of the population died of influenza.[44] This estimate is probably exaggerated, but the death rate was assuredly high. No separate figures for the plantation population exist, but there is no reason to believe that the workers suffered any less than the general population. In addition the plantation recruits suffered heavily from dysentery and pneumonia before the influenza onslaught. Dysentery, pneumonia, and a variety of other ailments combined to bring about an intolerable death rate among recruits from the grassland divisions (Bamenda and Chang) and this disaster led to the cessation of all recruiting by political officers. After the 1918 disaster, labor became free and voluntary in fact as well as in official statements.

An analysis of the mortality figures for 1918 provides evidence of the causes of the high death rates during the German period, and a description of changes in the plantation system during and after 1918 indicates why the mortality rate never again became so terribly high. Official reports indicate that 94 Bamenda recruits and 129 Chang recruits died at the plantations during the year.[45] However, many more died during the trek. A gang of ten Bamundum workers was sent from Bamenda in April, but only five of them arrived at the plantations; one died en route, and four were left along the way due to illness.[46] Plantation officials complained about the weak and sickly condition of many of the laborers upon their arrival at the work sites.[47] Complaints were also made about the condition of the workers at the time of their dismissal and return to their homelands. An army officer stationed in Victoria described the appearance of a gang just dismissed:

They passed along the main road from Bota to Victoria, and in numerous cases were so emaciated, suffering from various diseases, and therefore in such a state of health, that many were unable to walk for more than, roughly, without exaggeration, a hundred yards at a stretch. . . . I was given to understand that their Towns were in more than on[e] instance over 100 miles distant. This, to my mind would mean that they would simply die in the road.[48]

In a gang of 38 Babungo workers, three died at the plantations and two on the way home.[49] This was not entirely the fault of the plantation managers. The Manager of Bibundi claimed that he had advised seven men in a gang of 78 to report to the hospital prior to their departure from the estate, but they refused and left for home.[50]

The number of trek deaths cannot be determined and thus the total number of deaths caused by migration to the plantations is uncertain. A report by the Assistant District Officer (A.D.O.) in Chang, however, suggests the magnitude of mortality. He noted that the official records showed 133 deaths in 1918 among the 1,879 recruits sent from Chang, but his investigations indicated that a total of 377 had died from the time the gangs left home and until they returned. The official death rate was 70.78 per thousand but, according to the Chang data, it was 200.64 per thousand. The A.D.O. remarked that for workers whose homes were in climatic areas similar to those of the plantations, the death rate was 16 percent, but for those with grassland origins a rate of 50 percent or more per village occurred.[51] Based on the official statistics, the death rate for recruited workers of Bamenda origin was 43.62 per thousand in 1918. We lack sufficient information upon which to determine an overall mortality rate including trek deaths. Nevertheless, each of the death rates calculated above is greater than the standard of 40 per thousand by which we judged the German period.

The unusual number of deaths stimulated several investigations. The information available relates only to recruited workers from Bamenda and Chang Divisions, that is, the workers from the grassland. There is no information on recruits from other areas or on voluntary workers. However, death rates among these two categories were apparently much lower than among grassland recruits.

Among the grassland workers at the plantations 223 deaths were reported. The major causes of these deaths were dysentery/diarrhea and pneumonia. Most of the deaths occurred at seaside plantations and particularly at Bibundi and Idenau (the Debundscha area). Although the evidence is not conclusive, the authorities seem to have tried to place grassland workers on plantations located inland and at higher locations. This suggests that the death rate among grassland workers stationed at the coast was extremely high. The major causes of death suggest that crowded living conditions and poor sanitation facilities were instrumental factors.

A government medical officer inspected several of the inland and higher elevation estates in mid-1918. He described sanitation conditions as "very bad" and housing as "in most instances bad." Eighty percent of the workers were anemic and 10 percent suffered from edema. Most men had contracted ankylostomiasis. Latrines were "irregularly shaped holes in the ground," full of human waste and mosquito larvae, and open to the elements. Often these were on hillsides near the camps and would overflow during rain storms. In many instances the workers did not bother to use the latrines.[52]

As the death rate increased, G. S. Podevin, District Officer in Bamenda, was ordered by the Resident to inspect the plantations and to make recommendations on how to improve conditions there. Podevin, who died later in the year of influenza, was a strong opponent of labor recruitment, and he had battled with the Plantation Department on many occasions to defend the

Table 3. *Causes of Deaths among Grassland Recruits, 1918, by Location of Plantation*

Cause	Seaside plantations	Inland plantations	Total
Ankylostomiasis	8	2	10
Bronchitis	7	2	9
Diarrhea	30	7	37
Dysentery	52	5	57
Influenza[a]	4[a]	23[a]	27[a]
Malaria	6	—	6
Oedema	12	—	12
Pneumonia	20	8	28
Other, cause identified[b]	21[b]	6[b]	27[b]
Unknown	10	0	10
Total	170	53	223

a. All influenza deaths occurred during the epidemic in November and December. Almost all grassland workers were stationed at inland plantations at that time.

b. Listed causes include abscess (5), beriberi (1), colic (2), epilepsy (3), hernia (1), rheumatism (2), and tetanus (1).

Source: File Qe/1918/9, p. 14.

interests of the workers he was ordered to recruit. His report was based on long experience with the situation as well as his mid-year tour of the plantations. He placed blame for the unfavorable conditions he found at the plantations on two factors: the failure of the Plantation Department to obey the labor laws then in effect, and the failure of the government to define the responsibilities of that department and the Political Department. He concluded:

It is mainly due to the fact that official supervision in the past has been non-existent that the present situation has arisen. . . . No amount of camouflage can disguise the fact that conditions as regards labour from the grassland country have been abominable and a scandal can no longer continue. Constant and adequate supervision and inspection is the only remedy.[53]

One of his several recommendations was put into effect immediately; no grassland-recruited labor was to work on plantations located at altitudes of less than 1000 feet. Podevin argued that assignment to the coastal locations had "been largely responsible for (the) abnormal death rate and physical deterioration" of the workers.[54]

There is some evidence that the death rate among voluntary workers was much lower than among recruits. During the ten-month period from January through October 1918, the manager of Molyko Estate, an inland plantation, reported only one death among his voluntary workers from Bamenda and Chang, and he employed on the average of 265 such workers per month. In contrast, during the single month of January, the only month for which data is available, six of 411 Chang recruits died.[55] On an annual basis the death rate of volunteer workers was 4.5 per thousand, but for the recruits it was 175.1 per thousand. These two groups had the same origins and were working on the same plantation, but apparently they suffered different mortality rates. Perhaps volunteer workers were healthier than recruits. Also, a volunteer was free to leave at will, but a recruit had to stay until the end of his contract. Thus, if a volunteer believed that a plantation was unhealthy for him, he could move on; the recruit could not. One other factor may be important. The manager of an inland plantation reported that his recruits were housed in the old German barracks, but that volunteers, who in some cases were accompanied by families, were allowed to live in separated dwellings ("huts"). The manager of Molyko stated that such "huts" were the major inducement for voluntary labor.[56]

Several factors seem to have been involved in the high death rates of 1918. Primary among these was the use of recruiting by political officers with the implicit threat of fine, imprisonment, and government harassment to back it up. Recruits from one climatic area, the interior highlands, were sent to another climatic area, the coastal lowlands. The recruits did not select their place of work, and, since they were on contract, they were not free to leave a site once assigned. Finally, the living conditions at the plantations were not conducive to the maintenance of good health—improper sanitation, inappropriate housing, inadequate food rations, and a lack of medical care. As far as can be determined there was only one medical doctor in the entire Victoria/Kumba Division in 1918 and his responsibilities went far beyond the care of plantation workers. The evidence indicates that very similar conditions had prevailed during the German period.

Changes in the plantation system were underway in 1918, but the disastrous mortality of that year caused the immediate implementation of certain reforms. Recruiting by political officers ended in September by order of the Resident,[57] an order which was later confirmed by the Secretary for the Southern Provinces.[58] The only form of recruiting that could continue was that by plantation managers. This did not have the force of government behind it and, therefore, all aspects of compulsion were lost. Also, the use of contracts was ended, so a worker could leave a plantation at will. The actions of the government now agreed with its policy, a situation confirmed in numerous letters and reports during subsequent years.[59]

Surprisingly, the free labor system after 1918 was capable of providing sufficient labor for the needs of the plantations. Even in 1919, the first year of a truly free labor system, the Resident in Buea remarked that "the supply of labour appears to be maintained without undue difficulty."[60] In 1924 the plantations were

sold to the former German owners, and in March 1925 direct
governmental management ended. The government stated that
the new owners must rely on good treatment of labor to insure
a sufficient supply of workers, for "it is not the function of Government to provide labour for private enterprise or to put any
pressure on the people to work for wages."[61] The report noted
that free labor had been successful for the past eight years, although the early attempts at recruited labor had to be abandoned
because of the adverse reaction of the population and because
recruitment had proved so injurious to their health. In almost
every year until the end of the period under consideration the
labor supply was reported to be satisfactory.

Other changes introduced in 1918 were retained in succeeding
years. The workers' dislike of the German barracks in which they
had been housed was obvious to many of the managers. During
the war some of the workers had moved out of the barracks and
constructed individual dwellings; and several estate managers
even paid laborers to construct such quarters. Eventually, a com-
promise appeared on most estates. Long, narrow buildings divided into six or more one-room quarters, built with cement
block or wood and with sheet metal or thatched roofs became
the most common mode of housing employees. In 1925 the Resident reported that two laborers (or one if he was with his
family) lived in each room.[62]

Sanitary conditions were also improved. Open holes as latrines,
or in one instance the use of a beach with high tides as a flushing
mechanism, were replaced by cement latrines with fly traps in
permanent buildings with roofs. Attempts were made to locate
latrines so that water supplies would not be contaminated and
pipe-borne water systems were installed in many locations.[63] A
system of inspection of housing and sanitation facilities by district
officers and health officers was instituted and plantation owners
were fined on several occasions for failure to meet sanitation
standards.

Medical care for the workers also improved. During the final
years of the war there had been a general shortage of medical
personnel in the Cameroons Province, no doctor being assigned

specifically to the care of plantation workers. Occasionally patients were transferred to government hospitals in Victoria or
Buea for treatment under the supervision of a physician, but
most laborers were treated in plantation hospitals by poorly
trained dressers. Some of these men were illiterate and a medical
doctor judged most of them incapable of determining the causes
of death of their patients.[64] After the return of the German owners, the plantation companies were required to employ physicians
and to provide free medical treatment for all employees. Several
doctors were employed on a full-time basis, and government doctors were engaged by the plantations on a part-time basis. In
1927 one full-time doctor was employed by the plantation owners' organization; in 1935 there were four.[65]

In 1935 Mr. W. Benson of the International Labor Office inspected labor conditions in Nigeria and the Gold Coast. He
visited eleven plantations in the Cameroon portion of Nigeria
and reported quite favorably upon conditions. He noted that
detailed regulations on housing and sanitation had been issued
by the government, and that "the sanitary arrangements prescribed are being executed. . . . Housing conditions, on the
other hand, differ widely."[66] He believed that conditions on
Cameroon plantations were superior to those prevailing elsewhere in Nigeria and that government supervision was stricter in
Cameroon.[67] Reports by government officers in 1940 and 1941,
just after the end of the period under consideration, are generally
similar to Benson's comments. Medical and sanitary conditions
were considered satisfactory, but housing varied enormously
from one estate to another. However, by this time all barracks
had been abandoned.[68]

These changes in modes of labor recruitment, housing, sanitation, and medical care coincided with a lowering of death rates
among plantation workers. The data available are not complete;
for some years no information on numbers of deaths and/or
workers could be located. However, mortality rates for thirteen
years between 1919 and 1939 have been calculated. The rates
varied from 4.46 per thousand in 1935 to 8.69 per thousand in
1926.[69] There was a general, but very slight, declining trend

from 1919 until 1936. However, the mortality rate increased from 1936 until 1939. These last four years were years of rapid expansion in the size of the labor force (from 15,700 workers in 1935 to 25,000 in 1939, an increase of 59 percent) and this expansion may have overwhelmed the improvements in housing and sanitation, thus causing a reincrease in the mortality rate. Too, labor was in short supply during these years and, as the demand for workers became greater, less healthy individuals may have been accepted for employment. The year 1918, however, was the last in the history of the plantations in which tragically high death rates were reported.

After 1918 the major cause of death was pneumonia. Sixty-nine deaths are attributed to it in 1938. Although dysentery and diarrhea were reported as common illnesses, only in the last few years of the period, when the labor force expanded rapidly, was dysentery listed as an important cause of death. Throughout the 1930s accidents were a major cause of death. In addition to pneumonia and dysentery, other common illnesses were bronchitis, malaria, rheumatism, tropical ulcers, and yaws.[70]

In this chapter we have not considered all of the effects of the migratory labor system upon the health of the Cameroon people. The Bakweri, for example, forced off their lands and placed in reservations, are still considered to be a demoralized and dying people.[71] Plantation workers were and are considered to be a major cause of a high incidence of venereal disease among the population in the plantation environs.[72] And it is probable, especially in the years of high mortality rates, that returning laborers carried many communicable diseases to their home villages and to villages along the migration routes.

In summary, there is adequate evidence that migration to the plantations caused high rates of morbidity and mortality during the first 34 years of the existence of these plantations—the German period and the first years of the British administration. During the mandate period between the two world wars the general health of the laborers improved significantly with a corresponding drop in mortality rates. Basic changes in recruiting and housing occurred during this latter period, accompanied by equally important changes in sanitation and medical care. Not surprisingly, there is a correlation between these changes and the improvements in the health of the laborers on the plantations.

Notes

Research upon which this paper is based was supported by the Foreign Area Fellowship Program, the International Development Research Center at Indiana University, and the Institute of International Studies of the University of South Carolina. Portions of this paper were published in Hans Illi, ed., *Kamerun: Strukturen und Probleme der Sozio-Okonomischer Entwicklung* (Mainz: Hase und Koehler, 1974), pp. 181–236.

1. Harry R. Rudin, *Germans in the Cameroons, 1884–1914: A Case Study in Modern Imperialism* (New Haven, 1938), p. 248; also p. 222.

2. An English translation of the letter, dated 6 May 1884, is published in Shirley G. Ardener, *Eye-Witnesses to the Annexation of Cameroon, 1883–1887* (Buea, 1968), pp. 84–86. A copy in German is contained in H. P. Jaeck, "Die Deutsche Annexion," *Kamerun unter Deutscher Kolonial Herrschaft*, Helmuth Stoecker, ed. (Berlin, 1960), I, 92–95.

3. Erik Hallden, *The Culture Policy of the Basel Mission in the Cameroons, 1886–1905* (Uppsala, 1968), p. 94. Also see Marc Michel, "Les Plantations allemands du mont Cameroon, 1885–1914," *Revue francaise d'histoire d'outre-mer*, LVII, 207 (1969), 185; and S. J. Epale, "The Origins of the German Plantations," *Agrarian Capitalism in Western Cameroon, 1885–1975* (Buea, 1975), pp. 27–62.

4. Karen Hausen, *Deutsche Kolonialherrschaft in Afrika. Wirtschaftsinteressen und Kolonialverwaltung in Kamerun* (Zurich and Freiburg, 1970), pp. 220–24.

5. Rudin, *Germans in the Cameroons*, p. 249. These figures are quoted from *DENKSCHRIFTEN uber die Entwickelung der deutschen Schutzgebiete in Afrika und der Sudsee: 1912–1913*, pp. 82–83. Also see F. St. C. Stobart, "Notes on Various Matters Concerning German Administration in Buea and Victoria Districts," p. 6 in File Cf/1915/2. Stobart quotes these figures from the 1912–13 report of the German Governor of Kamerun. References to "Files" in these notes indicate the identifying number of files in the Buea branch of the Cameroon National Archives.

6. Whether the Bakweri were left enough land to survive has been a vexing problem. See Edwin Ardener, Shirley Ardener, and W. A. Warmington, *Plantation and Village in the Cameroons: Some Economic and Social Studies* (London, 1960), pp. 267–344; Great Britain, *Report by His Majesty's Government in the United Kingdom . . . to the General Assembly of the United Nations on the . . . Cameroons . . . for the Year 1949* [Hereafter referred to as *Annual Report, 1949*] (London, 1950), pp. 302–11; and *Annual Report, 1948*, p. 75

7. Michel, "Les plantations allemands," p. 198. See Max F. Dippold, "L'Image du Cameroun dans la litterature coloniale allemand," *Cahiers d'etudes africaines*, XIII, 1 (1973), 37–59. Also see J. P. Mannox, Manager of Molyko Plantation, to the Political Officer, Buea, 13 May 1915, File Cf/1915/2; the 1920 Molyko Plantation Report, File Qd/a 1920/97; and *Annual Report, Cameroons Province, 1931*, 12, File Ba/1931/3. Epale notes that the coastal peoples were accustomed to owning large numbers of slaves who did all of the menial work, and thus the slave-owners loathed such work and would not consider labor

on the plantations, "Origins of the German Plantations," pp. 52–55. Also see S. Epale, "The Mobilisation of Capital in a Rural Milieu," *Rural Africana* (forthcoming) for a discussion of Bakweri attitudes to plantation labor.

8. Adolf Rüger, "Die Entstehung und Lage der Arbeiterklasse unter dem deutschen Kolonial Regime in Kamerun (1895–1905)," *Kamerun unter deuischer Kolonial Herrschaft*, Helmuth Stoecker, ed. (Berlin, 1960), I, 181. Also see Rudin, *Germans in the Cameroons*, p. 319; and Hallden, *Policy of the Basel Mission*, p. 98.

9. After his expedition of 1889, Zintgraff reported that Bali would provide a source of manpower less expensive than Monrovia and Accra and more secure than areas under British control. Elizabeth M. Chilver, "Paramountcy and Protection in the Cameroons: The Bali and the Germans, 1889–1913," *Britain and Germany in Africa*, P. Gifford and W. R. Louis, eds. (New Haven, 1967), p. 484.

10. This is considered in Hella Winkler, "Das Kameruner Proletariat, 1906–1914," *Kamerun unter Deutscher Kolonial Herrschaft*, H. Stoecker, ed. (Berlin, 1960), I, 251.

11. The competition between traders and planters is discussed in detail by Rudin, *Germans in the Cameroons*, pp. 315–37 and in Epale, "Origins of the German Plantations," pp. 28, 39, 57–58.

12. A summary and discussion of German labor laws and recruiting are contained in Resident, Buea, "Notes on the Labour Problem on the Plantations," 12 August 1961 in File Qd/a 1916/22.

13. Rudin, *Germans in the Cameroons*, pp. 320–22. Copies of some of these treaties may be seen in *Kolonial-Gesetzgebung*, XII, doc. 205. Also see Rüger, "Die Entstehung und Lage der Arbeiterklasse," pp. 194–99; and Chilver, "The Bali and the Germans," p. 495.

14. Rüger, "Die Entstehung und Lage der Arbeiterklasse," pp. 206–7; and Rudin, *Germans in the Cameroons*, pp. 321, 325, and 338–45.

15. Resident, Buea, "Notes on the Labour Problem."

16. Heinrich Schnee, *German Colonization Past and Future: The Truth about German Colonies* (London, 1926), p. 139. For an opposite point of view, see Great Britain, Foreign Office, Historical Section, *Treatment of Natives in the German Colonies* (London, 1920). [Handbooks, 114.]

17. The relationship between change in altitude and risk of disease for Ethiopian migrant workers is discussed in Robert W. Roundy, "Altitudinal Mobility and Disease Hazards for Ethiopian Populations," *Economic Geography*, LII, 2 (1976), 103–15.

18. R. E. Dumett, "The Campaign against Malaria and the Expansion of Scientific Medical and Sanitary Services in British West Africa," *African Historical Studies*, I, 2 (1968), 153. According to Buchanan and Pugh, the coast is tsetse infested, but the higher parts of the Cameroons are fly-free: *Land and People in Nigeria*, pp. 46–49.

19. *Annual Report, 1949*, p. 293.

20. Numerous descriptions of these quarters are available. See the "Annual Report for Victoria Farms, 1920" contained in File Qd/a 1920/97; Manager of Meanja Plantation to the Deputy Supervisor of Plantations, 9 December 1918, File Qd/a 1918/55; Resident, Buea, "Notes on the Labour Problem," File Qd/a 1916/22; and F. St. C. Stobart in African (West), No. 1039. *Reports on Various Matters Relating to the Cameroons*, 26, File Ba/1916/3.

21. Robert R. Kuczynski, *The Cameroons and Togoland: A Demographic Study* (London, 1939), p. 53.

22. Charles C. Hughes and John M. Hunter, "Disease and 'Development' in Africa," *Social Science and Medicine*, III (1970), 451.

23. Kuczynski, *The Cameroons and Togoland*, pp. 52–53, 58; also see Rudin, *Germans in the Cameroons*, p. 328.

24. W. F. Gowers, "The German Administration of the Cameroons," p. 46 in African (West), No. 1039. *Reports on Various Matters Relating to the Cameroons*, File Ba/1916/3. Also see the "Bamenda Division, Annual Report," p. 29, File Ba/1920/4.

25. Rudin, *Germans in the Cameroons*, pp. 322, 347.

26. George W. Barclay, *Techniques of Population Analysis* (New York, 1958), p. 134. Barclay's perceptive chapter, "The Study of Mortality," pp. 123–66, considers the problems encountered in analyzing these data.

27. Quoted in Chilver, "The Bali and the Germans," p. 510. Also see Rudin, *Germans in the Cameroons*, pp. 327–28.

28. As quoted in Gowers, "German Administration," p. 47.

29. *Ibid.*, p. 48.

30. File Aa/1918/38.

31. Sir Bryan Sharwood Smith, *Recollections of British Administration in the Cameroons and Northern Nigeria 1921–1957: "But Always as Friends"* (Durham, N.C., 1969), p. 24.

32. Schnee, *German Colonization*, p. 140. But also see Jean K. MacKenzie, *Black Sheep* (Boston, 1916), pp. 83–84.

33. See, for examples, Gowers, "German Administration," p. 46; and Stobart, "Notes on Various Matters," p. 7.

34. Stobart, Political Officer in Buea to the Chief Political Officer, Duala, 15 July 1915, File Cf/1915/2, and a letter from the Director of Plantations, Bota, dated 26 April 1916, File Qd/a 1916/3.

35. Resident, Buea, to District Officer, Ossidinge Division, 19 May 1916, File Qd/a 1916/16.

36. F. G. Lugard, "Comments on the Plantations Yearly Report for 1916," 11 November 1917, File Qd/a 1917/1. For similar comments see Political Advisor's Office, Duala, to Political Officer, Buea, 24 May 1915, File Cf/1915/2.

37. District Officer, Bamenda, to Resident, Buea, 28 January 1918, File Qe/1918/6. Recruiting procedures are described in a letter from the District Officer, Victoria Division, to the Supervisor of Plantations, 6 September 1916, File Qd/a 1916/22.

38. District Officer, Victoria, to the Chiefs of Ngolo, Batanga, Balondo, etc., June 1917, File Qe/1917/2.

39. Assistant District Officer, Kumba, to Resident, Buea, 26 June 1917, File Qe/1917/2. See District Officer, Kumba, to Resident, Buea, 21 May 1918, File Qe/1918/4, and Divisional Officer, Ossidinge, to the Resident, 8 June 1918, File Qe/1918/3.

40. Resident, "Notes on the Labour Problem on the Plantations," 12 August 1916, File Qd/a 1916/22.

41. Recruiting information for 1918 is in Files Qe/1917/2, Qe/1918/2, Qe/1918/3 and Qe/1918/6.

42. See File Qe/1918/4.

43. See the reports of G. S. Podevin, District Officer, Bamenda, File Qe/1918/9; and the District Officer, Chang, File Qe/1918/2.

44. "Provincial Half Yearly Report," p. 1 in File Bb/1919/1.

45. File Qd/a 1916/16.

46. Resident, Buea, to Supervisor of Plantations, 2 May 1918, File Qe/1918/6.

47. Acting Supervisor of Plantations to Resident, Buea, 10 May 1919, File Qe/1918/2. Also see Manager, Ekona Plantation to Deputy Supervisor of Plantations, 7 December 1918, File Qd/a 1918/55. The Resident reported, however,

that he had seen a gang of recruits, "strong, healthy looking men," Resident, Buea, to District Officer, Bamenda, 28 December 1917, File Qe/1918/6.

48. B. C. Chiswick, 3rd. Nigeria Regiment, Victoria, to District Officer, Buea, 12 July 1918, File Qe/1918/9.

49. Resident, Buea, to Supervisor of Plantations, 2 May 1918, File Qe/1918/6; and "Medical Department Report on Plantations in the Buea District," 21 October 1918, p. 2, File Qd/a 1918/55.

50. Manager of Bibundi Estate to Supervisor of Plantations, Bota, 12 September 1918, File Qd/a 1916/16.

51. Assistant District Officer, Chang, to Resident, Buea, 6 November 1919, File Qe/1918/2.

52. File Qd/a 1916/16.

53. File Qd/a 1918/55, "Medical Department Report on Plantations in the Buea District." Strongly worded rebuttals from various plantation managers are also contained in this file.

54. *Ibid.*, p. 4.

55. "Molyko Estate, Monthly Hospital Return, 1918," File Qd/a 1918/55.

56. Manager, Mukonje Estate, to Deputy Supervisor of Plantations, 12 December 1918; and Manager, Molyko Estate, to Deputy Supervisor of Plantations, 6 December 1918, File Qd/a 1918/55.

57. Resident, Buea, to Supervisor of Plantations, 9 September 1918, File Qe/1915/5; and telegrams, Resident, Buea, to all District Officers, 9–12 September 1918, File Qe/1918/2.

58. Secretary of Southern Provinces to Resident, Buea, 7 February 1919, File Qe/1918/2.

59. See "Bamenda Division Annual Report for 1918," p. 13, File Cb/1918/1; "Handing-Over Notes, Mr. P. V. Young, Resident, Buea, to Captain W. G. Ambrose," 28 January 1919, p. 2; "Handing-Over Notes, Dr. J. C. Maxwell, Resident, Buea, to Mr. J. Davidson," December 1919, p. 4; "Handing-Over Notes, Mr. W. E. Hunt, Resident, Buea, to Mr. E. J. Arnett," 12 November 1925, pp. 7–8, File Gc/1917/1; *Annual Report, 1926*, p. 48; and *Annual Report, 1929*, p. 138.

60. "Provincial Annual Report, 1919," p. 17, File Ba/1919/1. Also see "Annual Report, Cameroons Province, 1920," p. 48, File Ba/1920/4.

61. "Report to the League of Nations, 1925," p. 15, File Ba/1925/4. Also see "Cameroons Province, Annual Report, 1925," p. 4, File Ba/1925/1.

62. Resident, Buea, to Secretary, Southern Provinces, 30 November 1925, File Qe/1933/3. Also see Pleass, "Report on Labour Conditions in Victoria Division for the Year 1940," p. 4, File Qe/1929/1.

63. See "Kumba Division, League of Nations Report, 1936," p. 17, File Cd/1936/1. Also see the analyses of plantation inspections contained in most of the *Annual Reports*.

64. Medical Officer, Victoria, to Senior Resident, Buea, 2 December 1925, File Qe/1933/3.

65. *Annual Report, 1927*, p. 70; and *Annual Report, 1935*, p. 69.

66. W. Benson, "Report . . . on a Mission to British West African Dependencies," p. 2, File Qe/1935/3.

67. *Ibid.*, pp. 6–7.

68. Pleass, "Report on Labour Conditions," pp. 3–5, and "Report from Resident, Cameroons Province, to Secretary, Eastern Provinces," 6 February 1941, File Qe/1929/1.

69. The actual death rates of laborers may be slightly lower. In several cases deaths of laborers' dependents who were treated in plantation hospitals are in-

cluded in the mortality data. However, the number of dependents present on the estates is not included in the number of employees.

70. "Analysis of Prevalent Diseases in the Plantations, January to June, 1923," File Qd/a 1923/121. Discussions of health conditions, mortality, and morbidity rates are contained in most of the *Annual Reports.* More detailed information is found in some instances in the annual divisional and Cameroons Province reports. See, for examples, File Ba/1939/3 and File Cd/1934/1.

71. See the detailed study by Edwin Ardener, *Divorce and Fertility* (London, 1962). Also see B. T. Nasah, M. A. N. Azefor, and B. N. Ondoa, "Socio-Cultural Aspects of Fertility in Cameroon," *Sub-Fertility and Infertility in Africa,* B. K. Adadevoh, ed. (Ibadan, 1974), pp. 65–68.

72. The 1949 health survey found a 4.12 percent incidence of gonorrhea in Bafut, located far from the plantations, but incidences of 13.1 percent in Eastern Balong and 10.4 percent in the North West Area of Kumba Division, both near the plantations, *Annual Report, 1949,* p. 293. In 1948 an incidence of 21 percent for gonorrhea was found in Muea, a village located in the heart of the plantation district, *Annual Report, 1948,* p. 115. See "Inspection of Labour: Report for the Cameroons Province, 1940," File Qe/1929/1.

7

Increased Intercommunication and Epidemic Disease in Early Colonial Ashanti

James W. Brown

Many areas of Africa experienced serious epidemic disease in the late nineteenth and early twentieth centuries, a phenomenon generally attributed to the breakdown of relative isolation and the spread of disease through increased intercommunication.[1] New diseases were introduced and familiar diseases spread more rapidly. Two types of increased contact were involved: between disease environments within Africa which had previously been isolated from each other, and between Africans and non-Africans. Both types of contact increased the possibility of epidemics.

Ashanti,[2] however, experienced relatively few epidemics during the early colonial period (or later), and, except for influenza, none that was especially devastating. A likely explanation would be that Ashanti was less isolated compared with other areas of Africa in the precolonial period, and hence the earlier introduction of disease there resulted in the earlier development of immunities. A second possibility is that during the early colonial period European medical knowledge was more extensively applied in Ashanti than in other areas of Africa. This chapter examines these possible explanations in relation to the various epidemics that occurred in Ashanti during the first 35 years of colonialism.

The Isolation Factor

In the second half of the nineteenth century the Asante kingdom centered on the forest zone of modern Ghana, covering the area between approximately 55 miles and 235 miles inland, its capital, Kumasi, being some 120 miles from the coast. The Asante Confederation had coalesced in the early eighteenth century, and had expanded militarily through the early nineteenth century. An important motive for expansion was the Asante desire to control the major arteries of trade. Sitting astride the trade routes between the savanna to the north and the coast to the south, the empire increasingly directed the commerce flowing between the two through her own capital.

The combination of military and commercial contacts with both south and north ensured that Asante was by no means isolated from her African neighbors and from any diseases that might be peculiar to them. Relations with the north meant contact with a different ecological zone, the savanna, and its diseases. The south was primarily within the same West African forest environment as Asante, but the coast had substantial contacts with Europeans and their diseases. From the late fifteenth century the Gold Coast, to the south of Asante, was a major area of European commerce and residence. At various times there were as many as 46 different European forts and outposts along the coast.[3]

Coastal commerce involved the travel of Asante traders to the south and coastal (primarily Fante) traders to Kumasi. During the earlier part of the nineteenth century at least, individual Asante were not encouraged to trade and were usually not inclined to do so.[4] However, after the Asante defeat of 1874, the number of Asante going to the coast to trade increased as a result of the Asante government's reduced ability to control trade within the empire and because of changing attitudes toward commerce. The number of individuals moving from one area into another at any one time could be quite large. In one recorded instance, during disturbances in 1886, a group of some 150 Asante traders were murdered on their way to the coast.[5]

Commercial contacts were the most frequent and consistent, but Asante's military expeditions in the south during the nineteenth century involved a far greater concentration of individuals. Asante armies invaded the coast in 1806–7, periodically thereafter until 1816, then again in 1823–26, 1852 (without fighting), 1863, and 1874. The Asante force defeated at the battle of Katamanso in 1826 may have numbered as many as 40,000.[6]

Asante relations with the north were equally important. Commercial contact, especially the kola nut trade with the northeast, increased significantly during the nineteenth century. However, relatively few merchants moved between the savanna and Asante because royal policy during much of the nineteenth century restricted the major entrepots for trade with the north to the edge of the savanna, outside of Asante proper.[7] On the other hand, slaves from the north were a major item for which the kola was exchanged, and this meant a continual influx of possible disease-carriers who became resident in Asante and were not merely transient traders. Furthermore, although traders from outside the empire were severely restricted in their access to Asante, northerners from the savanna areas within the Asante empire, such as Gonja and Dagomba, had greater freedom of movement. Throughout the nineteenth century there was a community of northerners in Kumasi and probably in major provincial centers as well. Military contact with the north also continued during the nineteenth century, though more often for the purpose of putting down rebellion than extending the empire.

Not surprisingly, information on disease in precolonial Asante is spotty. Few Europeans visited precolonial Asante, and until late in the nineteenth century their visits were confined to the capital and the road to it. Somewhat ironically the most complete medical statement on precolonial Asante comes from one of the earliest European missions. Tedlie, the medical attendant who accompanied the Bowdich mission in 1817, reported that the most common diseases in Asante were "the Lues, Yaws, Itch, Ulcers, Scald-heads, and griping pains in the bowels."[8]

The only epidemic diseases noted in early records were venereal disease and smallpox. Tedlie is the only source on venereal disease, reporting two cases of gonorrhea and numerous cases of syphilis.[9] Both diseases were presumably endemic by the nineteenth century; they were well established in the first quarter of the twentieth.[10]

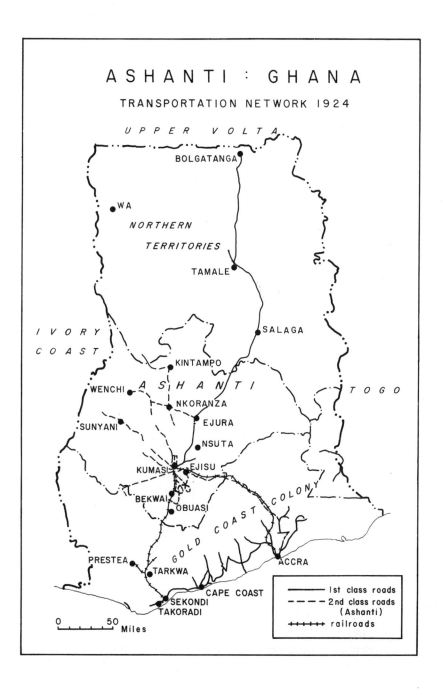

ASHANTI : GHANA

TRANSPORTATION NETWORK 1924

UPPER VOLTA

BOLGATANGA

WA

NORTHERN

TERRITORIES

TAMALE

IVORY
COAST

SALAGA

KINTAMPO

ASHANTI

TOGO

WENCHI

NKORANZA

EJURA

SUNYANI

NSUTA

KUMASI EJISU

BEKWAI

OBUASI

GOLD COAST COLONY

PRESTEA

TARKWA

ACCRA

CAPE COAST

SEKONDI
TAKORADI

	1st class roads
	2nd class roads (Ashanti)
	railroads

0   50
Miles

Smallpox had been noted on the coast at least as early as the seventeenth century, and in 1807 the first major Asante invasion of the coast was ravaged by the disease. It was also present in savanna West Africa from at least the early nineteenth century, and probably much earlier.[11] The Bowdich mission of 1817 recorded not only the presence of smallpox but the Asante method of inoculation against it: "They take the matter, and puncture the patient in seven places, both on the arms and legs. The sickness continues but a few days, and rarely any person dies of it."[12] Smallpox is the one epidemic disease whose presence in precolonial Asante produced immunities and indigenous forms of treatment sufficient to limit deaths during the subsequent colonial period.

Compared to the pre-Columbian New World or much of the rest of Africa, especially the interior of East and Central Africa, precolonial Asante was not isolated. It is not clear, however, that this lesser isolation was very important. For, while the presence of smallpox is certainly significant, smallpox was also common to many West African societies far more isolated than Asante. On the basis of present evidence, it would be difficult to conclude that Asante's lesser isolation during the precolonial period was a significant factor in reducing death by epidemic disease during the early colonial period.

Asante's contacts with the outside world greatly increased with the initiation of colonialism. The most obvious change was the entry of small numbers of European officials, missionaries, and merchants.[13] They concentrated primarily in Kumasi, the main administrative center, secondarily in the gold mining town of Obuasi, with the total in Ashanti averaging 259 by 1905.[14] Following closely behind the Europeans came Lebanese traders. Though the Lebanese also concentrated in the major commercial centers, they were much less confined to the towns, and some could be found following periodic market cycles in far more remote parts than ever saw European commercial men.[15]

Simultaneously, contacts with other Africans were accelerating. Asante policy had limited non-Asante commercial access to the empire, but under British ideas of free trade and access the number of African traders coming from both south and north grew. Northerners were especially prominent in the kola and cattle trades, with cattle replacing slaves as the major import from the north. The southerners continued their traditional trade in dried fish and European imports, but significant numbers of rubber brokers (buyers) from the south also spread out over the wild rubber producing areas of Ashanti, from which they had been excluded in the precolonial period.

In addition to traders there were also substantial numbers of coastal peoples and northerners lured to Ashanti by other employment opportunities. Southerners were especially attracted by the European demand for western-educated clerks, storekeepers, catechists, teachers, construction workers, and artisans. The influx was such that as late as the census of 1921 there were over half as many coastal peoples in Kumasi as there were Asante.[16] From the north migratory unskilled labor also flowed to the urban centers (northerners comprised some one-third of the population of Kumasi in 1921),[17] though most commonly they did seasonal agricultural work, especially after the rapid expansion of cocoa cultivation in the second decade of the twentieth century. New groups of Africans also arrived. Some, such as Sierra Leonean traders, were few, but there were also substantial numbers of such non-Gold Coast peoples as the Kru from Liberia, brought in by the British as manual laborers and carriers.[18]

Another addition was the British military force stationed in Kumasi. The size of the garrison fluctuated, but in 1902 it averaged some 800 African troops.[19] The soldiers were, however, much less likely to introduce epidemic disease than the civilian population, for they received relatively good medical attention. Indeed, during the early years, they and the government-employed clerks were virtually the only Africans to receive European medical treatment.

Thus, from the very beginning of the colonial period, the non-Asante presence in Ashanti increased substantially, and with it the increased possibility of the introduction of epidemic disease. Potentially counterbalancing elements of decreased intercommunication were few. They included the cessation of Asante military expeditions and the British-enforced halt to the flow of slaves from the north. Movement of Asante traders outside of Ashanti also decreased, for after the railway arrived in Kumasi in 1903 traders no longer needed to go to the coast for European manufactures, and they found themselves gradually excluded from the northern trade. Furthermore, especially with the development of cocoa, economic opportunities were readily available within Ashanti. Still, any decrease in contact as a result of less Asante movement outside Ashanti was more than counterbalanced by the greatly increased influx of non-Asante.

Intercommunication increased steadily with the continuing expansion of the transportation network. Because of Ashanti's potential cocoa wealth, its transportation infrastructure was developed much more extensively than in many other areas of Africa. The railroad was followed by motor roads, whose extent became significant during the second decade of the twentieth century. Each expansion of the road network made it economical to produce cocoa in still more areas—which meant more brokers and traders—while the roads themselves increased accessibility for administrators, catechists, relatives, and others. And as movement became easier, Asante farmers were more likely to go to the commercial centers to sell their cocoa and to spend their growing income. Growing numbers of Asante were therefore brought into contact not only with non-Asante, but also with other Asante, as improved transportation facilitated movement within Ashanti. And, clearly, this breakdown of microenvironments meant a greater likelihood that any active epidemic disease would spread more extensively.

The rapid growth of the transportation network, which generally provided a fairly immediate financial return through increased economic activity and customs duties for the government, was by no means matched by a comparable expansion of medical services. Further, the limited health care provided was heavily concentrated in the major towns. In 1921 there were only six medical officers in Ashanti. One of these worked with the miners at Obuasi, another was a temporary addition assigned to the railway construction, and two were in Kumasi, leaving one each for the provincial centers of Sunyani and Kintampo.[20] The census of 1921 gave an Ashanti population of 407,000, meaning that the doctor/population ratio was approximately 1:67,800 or, excluding the mines and railway doctors, approximately 1:100,000. There were four government hospitals for Africans, one each at Kumasi, Obuasi, Sunyani, and Kintampo, as well as contagious diseases hospitals at Kumasi and Obuasi.[21]

Another possible factor, which is difficult to assess on the basis of present evidence, is relative nutrition. Improved nutrition reduces susceptibility to disease, and the Asante undoubtedly did experience improved nutrition during the early colonial period. The wealth of Ashanti considerably increased, most notably with the expansion of cocoa, and this meant more money for food purchases, especially meat. Protein consumption must have increased with the substantial increase in the importation of cattle and dried fish, both of which became increasingly popular items of the diet. Dried fish imports fluctuated with the year, but ran as high as 999 tons imported by rail in 1912.[22] Cattle became the major import item from the north, coming from as far as Timbuktu. By 1908 Ashanti was importing some 20,000 head of cattle and 80,000 sheep and goats. By 1915 every big village was said to be obtaining a fairly constant meat supply, represented the following year by imports of over 77,600 head of cattle and some 100,000 sheep and goats.[23]

Epidemic Disease in
Colonial Ashanti

The recorded epidemics to strike Ashanti during the first three decades of the twentieth century were smallpox, influenza, meningitis, plague, and relapsing fever. Each of these epidemics is discussed below in chronological order, with summary and conclusions in the following section. In most cases the available material is seriously limited, and, with the exception of the information on the outbreak of plague in 1924, has not been greatly condensed for this paper. The epidemics discussed are the sig-

nificant recorded epidemics. Given the breakdown of micro-
ecologies discussed earlier, there may also have been epidemics
of such diseases as tuberculosis and venereal disease, but comparable information is not available.

The dependence on colonial records for data raises the question
of how accurately the disease situation among the African population can be described, especially in light of the concentration
of medical personnel in the major centers. This problem was especially serious in the very early years, when European administrators outside Kumasi were few and medical personnel were
concerned only with Europeans and soldiers. Even after the
Europeans became more widely distributed, mortality estimates
and other such figures remain highly suspect. It should not be
presumed, however, that European awareness of disease conditions among the African population, especially killing epidemics,
required the presence of medical officials. Any widespread epidemic affecting the adult male population would likely be noted
by political officers as part of their general responsibility. Outbreaks were especially significant in cash crop areas, where any
widespread epidemic among the adult male population would
affect economic productivity. Conversely, epidemics of childhood
diseases such as measles, which could result in serious population loss, might more easily go unrecognized or unrecorded. Indeed, there are no records of such epidemics, although some may
have occurred.[24]

The first recognized epidemic disease was smallpox. It is commented on as early as 1898 and again in 1901, when the European administration was still largely confined to Kumasi. The
1901 outbreak was undoubtedly an extension of the widespread
epidemic affecting the Gold Coast Colony at the same time.[25]
The disease was present throughout 1901, though it showed signs
of abating by the end of the year. The smallpox hospital in
Kumasi had only two patients at the end of December, but no
mention is made of the number treated during the year. The
medical officer reporting was unaware of any patients having
died, and no suggestion is given of a possible death rate among
those not committed to hospital.[26]

For smallpox, a possible counterbalancing effect of increased intercommunication would be the introduction of vaccination. The first mention of vaccination in Ashanti was during the last six months of 1905, with the vaccination of 1,361 Africans, primarily the soldiers and their wives and families.[27] In 1906 vaccinations were declared a failure. The vaccine was the lymph variety, which lost its potency in tropical conditions despite having been brought from Europe on ice. Though vaccine was subsequently prepared in Accra from 1911 to 1913, it was not much more effective, and consistently potent vaccine remained a problem, especially when it could not be kept cool. Not until 1957 did dried vaccine become common for use in the rural areas.[28]

After 1906 it was customary to report the successful vaccinations along with the total number, but Scott states that the usual 80–90 percent success rate reported was greatly inflated. In 1930, for the Gold Coast as a whole, the efficacy was more likely only about 20 percent.[29] Whatever the actual success rate may have been, the number of vaccinations increased over the years. By the fiscal year 1922–23 some 28,000 vaccinations were performed in Ashanti, some 18,000 (64 percent) being reported successful.[30]

The next smallpox epidemic, beginning in 1908, was introduced into Ashanti by northern migrants. It had been brought into the Northern Territories by Mossi from Upper Volta, and from there introduced into Ashanti. During 1909 it spread along the main trade routes, and then into the villages along the connecting paths, continuing throughout the next year and the first quarter of 1911.[31] Dr. Jupe, a European medical officer who traveled extensively in Ashanti performing vaccinations, noted that when the disease was introduced into a village, generally only the immune escaped. Case mortality varied from 15 percent to 40 percent, but he hazarded no guess on total mortality.[32]

Jupe traveled over 600 miles and estimated that he performed nearly 5,000 vaccinations with a success rate ranging from 3 percent to 100 percent, depending primarily on the freshness of the vaccine. He reported that the failure of old vaccine resulted in loss of prestige, but his reception was generally very cordial and most people desired vaccination. An increased vaccination effort continued throughout the epidemic, with the Asante willingly presenting themselves: in 1910, in the capital alone, 2,881 were vaccinated. In 1911 an African public vaccinator was appointed to travel through Ashanti; his success rate was estimated at approximately two-thirds.[33]

The Asante also continued to practice their traditional method of prevention, which Jupe described as the inoculation of the healthy from a pustule of a person with the disease. No attempt seemed to be made to choose a mild case. Jupe felt that this procedure usually produced a mild infection, though he also knew of several deaths resulting from such action and in one case was able to trace the introduction of smallpox into a village by inoculated individuals. The Senior Medical Officer in Ashanti suggested that this means of inoculation was serving to keep the disease alive, and the Chief Commissioner ordered that anyone except the medical officer who vaccinated for smallpox would be prosecuted under the criminal code.[34] The ruling is unlikely to have had much effect—probably none in villages away from major European administrative centers.

Figures on mortality during this epidemic are virtually nonexistent. The chiefs and people were unwilling to give the authorities any information on deaths, and the Europeans were aware of only a small percentage of cases. In the last four months of the epidemic, in early 1911, 37 cases were treated in the contagious hospital at Kumasi, with 11 deaths.[35]

The introduction of the disease from Upper Volta and its spread along the major trade routes indicate the significance of increased contact. Given the absence of reliable statistics on successful vaccinations as a percentage of total population, it is much more difficult to assess the role of the colonial medical service in containing the disease. Though the European presence may have somewhat mitigated the potential severity, it clearly was insufficient to halt the advance of the epidemic, which took over three years to run its course. It should also be noted that previously established immunities and the practice of traditional inoculation were also insufficient to stop the epidemic.

By far the most devastating disease to strike Ashanti was the pandemic of "Spanish" influenza in 1918. The records indicate this and my African informants were agreed that no other outbreak of disease was remotely as serious.[36] The epidemic began in Europe in 1918. The first train load of returning soldiers arrived in Kumasi on 8 September; by 17 September alarming accounts of the spread of the disease were current, and there were several soldiers in hospital with what was feared might be the "flu." The first confirmed case was on 23 September, and the same day the government closed schools and attempted to prevent assemblages of any kind. The Chief Commissioner of Ashanti suggested to the Governor that railway travel should be restricted, but was informed that elsewhere it had proved impossible to exclude the epidemic and the only option was to let it run its course and provide as many medical facilities as possible. Serious efforts were made in Ashanti, however, with the confining of soldiers to their barracks and the eventual closing of major roads—though with no evidence of significant effect on the course of the disease.[37]

An extra hospital was opened in Kumasi on 3 October, but within a few days many of the African medical assistants were sick. At the gold fields in Obuasi nearly the entire African labor force bolted for their homes, three European miners died, and the mine was closed on 11 October. By 18 October the epidemic was reported spreading rapidly in the Nsuta Division, from which many miners came. But by that time the disease was advancing in many areas of Ashanti. For example, at the provincial center of Ejisu two-thirds of the population was affected. During the peak of the disease in a given area, most normal activity came to a virtual standstill.[38]

By the last week of October the disease was abating in Kumasi, with the known death rate down to six daily from a peak of about 20 a day. It was acknowledged, however, that official figures by no means represented the real loss sustained, for by far the greater portion of bodies were taken out of the town for burial in the natal village and remained unregistered. The disease lingered on in some districts until at least the second week in December.[39]

Obtaining mortality figures for Ashanti was obviously impossible, but the Chief Commissioner estimated a total of some 9,000 deaths, or about 2 percent of the population. Some districts suffered much more heavily than others. Central Province, focusing on Kumasi, was estimated to have accounted for 4,500 deaths, over half of the total. Southern Province, the location of Obuasi, accounted for another 2,500, with the remaining 2,000 divided between 1,500 in the Western Province and 500 in the Northern Province.[40] The reported severity of disease in the central and southern areas possibly reflected the greater European presence and awareness of conditions, combined with somewhat greater population, but this is also the area in which the transportation infrastructure was most extensively developed and movement of population greatest.

In Kumasi, where the most accurate statistics could be compiled, 388 registered deaths were attributed to influenza, including two Europeans and five Lebanese.[41] Since the majority of African deaths were felt to have gone unregistered, 800 would be a conservative estimate of African deaths. With an approximate population of 20,000,[42] this would mean a death rate of some 4 percent of the total African population of Kumasi. Such a figure would be somewhat above that for small groups for which fairly accurate figures are available. Of the 762 Africans in the regiment, 267 were attacked and 25 died (3.3 percent). Of 183 African employees of the government, 70 got influenza and 5 died (2.7 percent). In contrast, the 75 police suffered a 6.6 percent death rate.[43] These groups represent the Africans most likely to seek and receive European medical treatment, but little could be done to treat the disease except bed rest.

In light of the likely accuracy of the figure of 25 deaths in the regiment, one might note the impression left on the mind of an informant who at that time held a high-level clerical position with the regiment. He stated that a big hole was dug for the soldiers and the dead bodies were packed in, with about 100 dying a day.[44] Clearly the influenza epidemic left a vivid impression on his memory, but his, and probably other informants' recollections of figures must be examined with care.

The next major epidemic was cerebrospinal meningitis in 1920. This was an extension of an epidemic in the Northern Territories, and affected only some sections of northern Ashanti, areas that are now in the separate province of Brong-Ahafo. The Nkoranza district was most seriously affected, with over 70 deaths.[45]

Cerebrospinal meningitis is transmitted by aerial droplets. The meningococcus which causes the disease is very delicate, and epidemics usually occur only when there is serious overcrowding in poorly ventilated areas, especially sleeping quarters. In the savanna country of the north, this situation prevails, at least among the poor, during the season of the harmattan winds that blow off the Sahara during the first few months of each year. Such conditions do not prevail in most of Ashanti, and the spread of the disease to the south has generally been considered unlikely and has not occurred.[46]

The major roads in northern Ashanti were closed in an effort to contain the spread of the disease. The main roads leading into Kumasi from the affected areas were also cordoned off with troops, and everyone coming from the infected area was examined by a medical official.[47] No cases were reported in Ashanti outside the north, but no significant spread of the disease would be expected even without the imposed restrictions.

Plague broke out in Kumasi in April 1924. Plague is generally transmitted to humans by the bite of fleas that become carriers by feeding on infected rats. Once present in humans it can become pneumonic plague, which is conveyed from one person to another by aerial droplet infection.

Kumasi was almost certainly infected from the port of Sekondi, where a serious outbreak of plague began in early March. Kumasi was the inland terminus of the railroad from Sekondi, and 564 passengers as well as large quantities of goods suitable for flea and rat infestation arrived in Kumasi by train between 14 March and 8 May, while Sekondi was in quarantine. The goods shed serving the railroad in Kumasi was not far from several stores, including the rat-infested United Trading Company Store, where the first man in Kumasi to contract plague worked. He lived in the section of the town near the railroad goods shed, and it was in this section, between 1 April and 9 May, that seven of the first nine cases of plague occurred.[48]

Plague was thought to have been introduced into Sekondi by

a ship coming from Lagos, the Canary Islands, Portuguese or French West Africa. Lagos had a serious epidemic of plague at the time, the Canary Islands were also infected, and plague was thought to be endemic along the Ivory Coast. P. S. Selwyn-Clarke, Medical Officer of Health in Kumasi during much of the outbreak there, reported that epidemic plague often occurred in various areas of French West Africa, but he considered the introduction of the disease to Kumasi from such a source most unlikely, given the absence of any cases within a wide radius of the city.[49]

Whether plague had ever occurred previously in Kumasi or Ashanti is unclear. Selwyn-Clarke could find no evidence in the available European records of the prior existence of the disease in Kumasi or the surrounding area. The Asante population, on the other hand, felt that the disease was nothing new, and that they could treat it with traditional medicines.[50] An outbreak among humans usually follows an epizootic among rats. Such an epizootic seemed indicated in Kumasi by later clinical tests on rats that verified the presence of the disease even when the normal external symptoms were absent. This suggested that the disease had been present long enough for the rats to have acquired some immunity, though they were still carriers. It was unclear, however, how long it would have taken for such a condition to develop, and the medical authorities believed that the disease had not been present among the Asante of the Kumasi area prior to this outbreak.[51]

Nine deaths occurred between 1 April and 9 May, during which time the medical authorities attempted to combat the disease with some 2,000 antiplague vaccinations. After a lapse the plague reappeared in another part of the town, the Zongo Extension. The outbreak in this area was initially unknown to the medical and sanitary authorities. Between 28 May and 9 June seven men died in one compound, five of the deaths being concealed from the sanitary inspector at the time. The deaths were later presumed to be plague, for within the next six days three fatal cases of confirmed plague occurred in a compound some 20 yards away. The disease could not have been contracted outside

Kumasi, for all those who died had been resident in the city for a minimum of two months. Seemingly the only possible connection with the first cases was that some of the deceased were kola traders who had occasionally visited the railroad goods station in the area of the original outbreak. Whatever the source, Zongo Extension now became a new center for the disease's spread, and 48 cases subsequently occurred in the same area.

Because the cause of the initial known deaths in Zongo Extension was not immediately realized, no antiplague measures were at first instigated. The inability of the sanitary officials to keep abreast of conditions was scarcely surprising, given a general inclination among city residents not to report such information and the limited number of sanitary inspectors employed. The sanitary division at the time consisted of one European superintendent and seven African inspectors. An inspector was unable to check any one compound more than once every two or three weeks.

The appearance of the disease in the Zongo area was fateful. The Zongo and Zongo Extension comprised a large area of the town where the majority of Muslims from Nigeria and the immigrants from the Northern Territories and French West Africa lived. It was one of the poorest, least sanitary, and most overcrowded areas of Kumasi. The great majority of living and sleeping rooms had no source of light or ventilation, and the consequent damp darkness made ideal conditions for plague dissemination. In many cases animals were kept in the open compound yard and even in the living rooms. The fodder for these animals, especially corn for horses, created ideal conditions for rats. Some compounds were also used for wholesaling large quantities of various grains and agricultural commodities, which also attracted rats. Residences were overcrowded and close to each other, while sanitary facilities were virtually nonexistent.[52]

A number of the early plague victims in Zongo Extension had frequented the insanitary and rat-infested Zongo market, from which the disease seemingly spread to the Zongo proper and to Fanti New Town. Akan from the coastal areas were the major inhabitants of Fanti New Town, but they used the Zongo market because it was closer than the market that served most of the other Akan, including the Asante. Fanti New Town, unlike the Zongo area, was relatively new and prosperous with generally higher standards of construction and sanitation, and the outbreak was much less severe there. Later in the epidemic cases appeared in other parts of Kumasi, many of which were traceable to the Zongo and Zongo Extension. By this time, however, the anti-plague measures of the authorities were having some effect, aided by generally better sanitation in other areas of the town. Zongo and Zongo Extension accounted for over 80 percent of the total cases.

Several antiplague measures were undertaken. The major outbreak occurred between mid-June and mid-September 1924, during which time over 103,000 antiplague vaccinations were performed. After initial resistance, popular demand for vaccination generally exceeded the available supply. Though vaccination could not legally be required of everyone in the town, Kumasi was placed under quarantine, and no one could leave the town without a certificate of vaccination. The number of vaccinations, allowing for revaccinations, represents at least three times the population of Kumasi at the time, the additional numbers representing large numbers of residents of the surrounding villages and persons passing through this important commercial center.

Vaccination proved to be significant in combatting at least one of the varieties of plague present in Kumasi. Of the 140 cases proved bacteriologically to be plague during the period of quarantine, some 64 percent were bubonic plague, 19 percent pneumonic, and 17 percent septicaemic.[53] Of the 29 cases of primary and secondary pneumonic plague, 11 (38 percent) had been vaccinated prior to the incubation period, indicating that vaccination was ineffective against pneumonic plague. The situation with septicaemic plague was inconclusive, but of the 90 cases of bubonic plague, only six (6.7 percent) had been vaccinated prior to the incubation period. Thus vaccination seemingly did restrict the spread of the most prevalent variety of plague in Kumasi, bubonic.

When cases of plague were discovered, the dead were quickly

buried and the living were transported to the Contagious Diseases Hospital. A police guard was placed at a victim's residence, which was sealed and disinfected. All contacts living in the same residence (the number averaged 25) had their clothing disinfected, were vaccinated if they had not been previously, and were then confined for ten (later twelve) days. During this time they were examined daily by the Medical Officer of Health. Such restrictions on contacts undoubtedly helped limit the spread of the disease, but they also encouraged efforts to conceal cases or to remove victims from their original compounds, even though such actions were prosecuted where possible.

Over 6,800 rooms were disinfected with sulphur dioxide. This figure included all rooms in the Zongo and Zongo Extension, a number of which were done several times. Some 129 of the most insanitary residences, containing a total of 802 rooms, were demolished. Temporary accommodation was provided for a number of the dispossessed, some 1200 of whom were living in government-constructed permanent residences by March 1925.[54] In addition to demolition of whole residences, an effort was made to convince the entire town to demolish the verandahs and various structures cluttering originally open compound yards and to have at least two windows in every room. More than 3,000 new windows were constructed in the Zongo and Zongo Extension alone —sometimes after the forceful encouragement of having a hole knocked through the mud wall in the suggested location of a new window. In addition the entire Zongo market was cleared and two long, airy market sheds were constructed.

The effort to reduce conditions favorable to rat breeding also included the clearing of large areas of bush in and around the town and persuading horse owners in the Zongo to remove their animals from the residential area. To aid the latter effort, the Sarkin Zongo (the African head of the Zongo) built a stable for some 40 horses outside the town.

An average of 200 rat traps were set daily, the traps being ones that caught the rats alive so that the fleas would remain on them. Over 4900 rats were captured in this way, out of an estimated rat population of some 25,000 to 30,000.[55] Further, payment of

2d. was offered for every rat brought to the authorities, which yielded an additional 797. "KILL RATS AND STOP PLAGUE" or its equivalent in various African languages was whitewashed on structures throughout the town. Those failing to adopt antirat measures dictated by the sanitary authorities, such as filling rat holes and concreting floors, were subject to prosecution.[56]

All schools and the cinema were closed. No assemblies for funerals were permitted, nor for other social and religious gatherings, including the important Muslim celebrations connected with Ramadan. Churches, however, were permitted to continue services, for they were all well ventilated and it was hoped that the clergy would preach sanitation and antiplague measures from the pulpit. Many did.

These rigorous antiplague measures were seldom appreciated by the local population, who especially resented demolition of unauthorized structures and the demand for windows. Active support from the Sarkin Zongo, the African authority for the area of greatest plague incidence, was a great help in reducing tension among those most affected by antiplague measures. The Asante, however, who suffered only a few cases of plague, adopted a policy that amounted to virtual passive resistance.[57]

Appreciated or not, the antiplague campaign proved sufficient to contain the disease, which began to abate by mid-August.[58] By mid-September no new cases were being reported, and the quarantine was lifted. A brief new outbreak in mid-November resulted in the town's being again placed in quarantine for eleven days, after which only occasional cases occurred through March 1925. These brought the total to 166, with 145 deaths.[59] No significant incidence of plague occurred outside Kumasi, but suspicious cases always resulted in vigorous measures. For example, a possible case was reported in Bekwai the night of 27 December 1924. The town was visited the following morning, a general clean up was initiated, and over 9,000 antiplague vaccinations were given.[60]

The epidemic of plague spurred a significant improvement in the sanitary condition of Kumasi that naturally had beneficial effects on public health. In addition, specific antiplague measures were maintained for a number of years, directed at such things as rat-proofing of houses and stores and the capture of rats. The number caught had increased to over 24,500 by 1930–31.[61]

Plague was clearly introduced from outside Ashanti. It is unlikely that plague would have occurred in Ashanti at all without the improved transportation provided by the railroad. It seems equally clear that the rigorous application of western medical knowledge contained the epidemic. Thus by at least the mid-1920s the presence of the European colonial administration was having a significant effect in limiting the outbreaks of epidemic disease that increased intercommunication had made more likely.

A similar pattern is seen in the outbreak of relapsing fever in 1927. Louse-borne relapsing fever broke out in Kumasi in March 1927, resulting in 31 cases and two deaths. The disease was confined to those from the Northern Territories and may have been introduced from the French Sudan, which was experiencing a serious outbreak with heavy case mortality. The disease recurred in the latter half of 1927 with an additional 97 cases, five fatal, treated at the Contagious Diseases Hospital. Cases again occurred entirely among men from the Northern Territories. Many of these migrants came from areas much drier than the forests of the south, did not practice the regular bathing of the southern peoples, and generally harbored far more lice. Preventive measures consisted of the removal to the Contagious Disease Hospital of all known cases, which were usually found lying in the Zongo market in the morning. They were then deloused and treated.[62]

The fatal cases were all individuals in an acute stage of starvation. Many of the migrants from the Northern Territories were in a debilitated condition, having walked down from the north in search of work, especially during the cocoa season, and frequently arriving in such poor physical condition as to be unemployable. To deal with this situation the Kumasi Public Health Board in 1927 erected a hostel to provide accommodation, with the Sarkin Zongo providing food,[63] reducing though not preventing the introduction of contagious diseases from the north.

Another outbreak of relapsing fever among northern immigrants in Kumasi occurred in 1930–31 with 70 cases and three

deaths. In addition to measures adopted earlier, all known contacts of cases of relapsing fever were collected, deloused, and
isolated in the Contagious Diseases Hospital for ten days. All
lousy persons entering Kumasi by the North Road were bathed,
shaved, and had their clothes disinfected. A similar procedure
was used after periodic police round-ups of the group to which
the disease was confined. On the most notable occasion over
1,100 persons were cleaned in one day.[64]

One final epidemic should be noted; smallpox occurred in
1929–30 in the southern Ashanti mining center of Obuasi. The
disease was almost certainly an extension of the outbreak in the
nearby Gold Coast Colony. Vaccination accelerated, with large
numbers of the population coming forward. In Kumasi alone,
which was unaffected, some 121,825 vaccinations were performed, and the disease did not spread.[65] Previous immunity
combined with western medicine were seemingly responsible for
the limited incidence of the disease.

Conclusion

During the early colonial period Ashanti enjoyed a relative
absence of serious epidemics. Epidemic diseases were present,
but the death rates associated with them were considerably less
than those reported for some other areas of Africa. A lesser degree of isolation than much of the rest of Africa during the precolonial period would be only a partial and inadequate explanation. Asante was indeed less isolated, but the significance of this
greater contact for early introduction of disease is only clearly
demonstrated in the case of smallpox. The presence of smallpox
in Asante for an undetermined but considerable period meant the
presence of immunities and means of treatment and prevention
(inoculation) that lowered death rates from smallpox during the
early colonial period. The presence of smallpox, however, is
clearly not an adequate explanation for the relative absence of
other serious epidemics.

Increased intercommunication during the early colonial period made the introduction of disease from outside Ashanti more likely, and, once introduced, greatly facilitated the possible spread of infection. Indeed, given the great amount of intercommunication relative to many areas of Africa, the situation would seemingly have been ideal for the spread of epidemic disease. But given the lack of precolonial isolation, it would be very difficult to say that a given disease introduced during the colonial period resulted from the increase in intercommunication and would not have occurred at the levels of intercommunication prevailing earlier. Only with plague does a clear case seem to exist. Nonetheless, one must note that during the first 30 years of the twentieth century all major epidemics, with the possible exception of cerebrospinal meningitis, are apparently attributable to the introduction of disease from outside Ashanti. The outbreaks of smallpox began as extensions of epidemics outside Ashanti. Influenza was introduced by returning soldiers, though influenza was so worldwide in scope that it undoubtedly would have arrived eventually. The presence of plague in Kumasi was clearly the result of greater intercommunication, for it came from the coast by means of the railroad and was brought to the coast by ship. Relapsing fever was introduced into central Ashanti by migrant laborers from the north, whose greatly increased presence was one of the many aspects of growing contact with other areas. Increased movement within Ashanti seems especially significant in the spread of smallpox and influenza. Though Ashanti was not struck in the early colonial period by epidemics of the severity experienced in many areas of Africa, the incidence and extent of epidemic disease were greater because of increased intercommunication.

Not until the mid-1920s did the presence of European colonial rule, through rigorous application of western medical knowledge, contribute significantly to restricting the spread of epidemic diseases. This seems true for all three of the diseases of the mid and late 1920s—plague, relapsing fever, and smallpox—but is clearest in the case of plague. Plague might have caused many more deaths in Kumasi, and the large transient population of the town could have carried the disease much more widely. Relapsing

fever also occurred in Kumasi, but in this case dissemination outside the city would probably have been restricted to northerners
in Ashanti and not to the more lice-free Asante. Furthermore,
while Kumasi had a large transient population, it also had the
greatest concentration of colonial officials and medical personnel,
so it was possible to initiate a more rigorous attack on epidemic
disease there than in more remote areas. Similarly, the outbreak
of smallpox in Obuasi in 1929–30 occurred in a population center
with a large number of immigrants who could have spread the
disease, but it was also a center for Europeans, including medical
personnel for the mines.

Although the larger question of why there was not still greater
introduction and spread of disease in Ashanti during the early
colonial period is beyond the scope of this paper, a few thoughts
may be ventured. The factor of relative precolonial isolation, or
the lack thereof, was of limited significance for Asante. Much of
West Africa may not have varied significantly in degree of isolation. Smallpox was the most significant by-product of relative
nonisolation for Asante, but smallpox was widespread in precolonial West Africa. Though West Africa may not have varied
significantly in disease immunities by virtue of differences in
relative isolation, there were significant differences in the effects
of epidemic disease during the early twentieth century. Areas of
the savanna seem to have been more severely attacked, with
major epidemics of such diseases as relapsing fever, cerebrospinal
meningitis, and human trypanosomiasis.

Why Ashanti, and perhaps the forest area more generally, were
not so seriously affected will require extensive examination, but
relevant factors for future investigation include relative nutrition,
prosperity, availability of medical facilities, and medical capabilities. Another factor would be the effect of varying ecological
conditions and life styles on disease transmission. Among the diseases discussed here, cerebrospinal meningitis, because of its
mode of transmission, requires crowded living conditions which
generally do not exist in the ecological conditions of the forest.
Similarly, better sanitation in the Asante areas of Kumasi helped
reduce the rat population and restrict the spread of plague from

the Zongo to the Asante areas. As regards relapsing fever, the availability of water in the forest, an ecological factor, has undoubtedly influenced the development of a life style that includes frequent bathing, which reduces the number of body lice and limits transmission of louse-borne disease. Factors such as these, which go beyond the question of relative isolation and increased intercommunication, will need further examination before we have an adequate explanation of the relative absence of serious epidemics in Ashanti during the early colonial period.

Notes

The field research on which this chapter is partially based was funded by the Comparative World History Program of the University of Wisconsin and by the Danforth Foundation.

1. The literature is limited, but see for example Charles M. Good, "Salt, Trade, and Disease: Aspects of Development in Africa's Northern Great Lakes Region," *The International Journal of African Historical Studies,* V, 4 (1972), 543–86; David Scott, *Epidemic Disease in Ghana 1901–1960* (London, 1965); and Philip D. Curtin, "Epidemiology and the Slave Trade," *Political Science Quarterly,* LXXXIII, 2 (1968), 190–216.

2. As used here the term Ashanti designates the colonial administrative district of that name; the term Asante refers to the precolonial kingdom and the people.

3. W. E. F. Ward, *A History of Ghana,* 4th ed. rev. (London, 1967), pp. 434–39.

4. T. Edward Bowdich, *Mission from Cape Coast Castle to Ashantee,* ed. W. E. F. Ward, 3d. ed. (London, 1966 [1st. pub. 1819]), p. 395.

5. W. Walton Claridge, *A History of the Gold Coast and Ashanti from the Earliest Times to the Commencement of the Twentieth Century,* (London, 1964), II, 285.

6. Ivor Wilks, *Asante in the Nineteenth Century: The Structure and Evolution of a Political Order* (London, 1975), p. 183. The invasions of 1807, 1825, and 1873 were all eventually ravaged by smallpox and dysentery.

7. Ivor Wilks, "Asante Policy Towards the Hausa Trade in the Nineteenth Century," in *The Development of Indigenous Trade and Markets in West Africa,* ed. Claude Meillassoux (London, 1971), pp. 127–28; Wilks, *Asante in the Nineteenth Century,* pp. 267–71, 282–87.

8. Bowdich, *Mission to Ashantee,* p. 374.

9. *Ibid.,* pp. 377, 379. Given the possible confusion between syphilis and the common African disease yaws, both of which may have the same causative organism, it may be worth noting that Tedlie did distinguish between the two diseases.

10. G. R. Griffith, District Commissioner, Central Province Ashanti, to Chief Commissioner of Ashanti [hereafter CCA], 23 March 1915, ADM 51/4/48, National Archives of Ghana, Accra [hereafter NAG]; Report on Kumasi by Dr. O. G. Wilde, Medical Officer, 20 October 1925, CO/96/662, Public Records

Office, London [hereafter, PRO]. Venereal disease was placed at the top of the list of prevailing diseases among the Asante when a venereal clinic was opened in Kumasi in 1919 (*Colonial Reports*, Ashanti, 1919).

11. Kwamina B. Dickson, *A Historical Geography of Ghana* (Cambridge, U.K., 1969), p. 58; Eugenia W. Herbert, "Smallpox Inoculation in Africa," *Journal of African History*, XVI, 4 (1975), 543–44.

12. Bowdich, *Mission to Ashantee*, p. 409. The description is actually of the practice in the "Moorish countries," followed by the statement that "it is also done in Ashantee."

13. The last Europeans to have an extended residence in Kumasi were captured mission personnel held in Kumasi during the early 1870s.

14. *Colonial Reports*, Ashanti, 1905.

15. Interviews: H. S. Hany, Kumasi, 13 May 1970; Mrs. William Joseph, Kumasi, 18 May 1970; Ernest Mourkarzel, Kumasi, 20 May 1970; Ernest Mourkarzel, Kumasi, 30 May 1970.

16. Census Report, 1921, Form E, Tribes, comp. F. W. Applegate, Acting Police Magistrate, n.d., D/1589, National Archives of Ghana, Kumasi Branch [hereafter NAG/K].

17. *Ibid.*

18. As early as February 1896, the Foreman of Works in Kumasi had in his employ three gangs of Kru. Phillips to Governor, n.d., encl. in Governor Maxwell to Secretary of State, 3 March 1896, Colonial Office Print, No. 504, CO/879/44, PRO.

19. *Colonial Reports*, Ashanti, 1902.

20. *Colonial Reports*, Ashanti, 1921.

21. Kumasi had had various such centers since early in the century. Obuasi's opened in 1913. *Colonial Reports*, Ashanti, 1913.

22. *Colonial Reports*, Ashanti, 1912.

23. Of the 20,000 head of cattle imported in 1908 approximately 10 percent were exported to the Gold Coast by rail, 50 percent were consumed in the areas of Kumasi and Obuasi, and 40 percent went to the rest of Ashanti. The cattle and sheep imports of 1916 represented an estimated value of £410,000, of which £50,000 were exported to the Gold Coast. Trade Report for 1908, Ashanti, n.d. C/8, NAG/K; *Colonial Reports*, Ashanti, 1915 and 1916.

24. A possible exception is an outbreak of chicken pox in 1912, tersely described as "fairly prevalent," with 81 cases treated in Kumasi. (*Colonial Reports*, Ashanti, 1912). The report does not state or imply that such cases were not adults. If so, there presumably was not an immunity from childhood, and the disease may have been newly introduced as a result of increased intercommunication. The absence of further information makes it impossible to do more than speculate.

25. W. B. Thain, Senior Medical Officer, Health Report for Kumasi in the Ashanti Annual Report, 1901, ADM 5/1/78, NAG.

26. Scott, *Epidemic Disease*, p. 68.

27. *Departmental Reports*, Medical and Sanitary Report, 1905 and 1906.

28. Scott, *Epidemic Disease*, p. 83.

29. *Ibid.*, p. 82.

30. *Colonial Reports*, Ashanti, 1922–23.

31. These are the generalizations found in the records and not generalizations based on specific data found in the records. They thus do not lend themselves to more extensive analysis, such as diffusion models.

32. Dr. I. Jupe to CCA, 12 January 1910, C/248, NAG/K; Scott, *Epidemic Disease*, p. 68.

33. Dr. I. Jupe to CCA, 12 January 1910, C/248, NAG/K; *Colonial Reports, Ashanti*, 1910 and 1911; *Departmental Reports,* Report of the Medical and Sanitary Department, 1910.

34. Dr. I. Jupe to CCA, 12 January 1910, C/248, NAG/K; Griffith to Sgt. Mensah, 28 April 1910, SCT/201/4, NAG/K.

35. *Colonial Reports, Ashanti,* 1910 and 1911.

36. Interviews: Mercy Aggrey, Kumasi, 20 May 1970; Arnold Anderson Agbolosoo, Kumasi, 22 May 1970; Ewe, Kumasi, 8 April 1970; Kwadjo Mprah, alias Jacob Frimpong, Kumasi, 11 May 1970; Mrs. William Joseph, Kumasi, 18 May 1970; Toasehene Kofi Owusu, Kumasi, 13 May 1970.

37. Fuller, CCA, Diary, September, 1918, ADM/12/5/160, NAG; Interview, Toasehene Kofi Owusu, Kumasi, 13 May 1970.

38. Fuller, CCA, Diary, October, 1918, ADM/12/5/142, NAG.

39. Fuller, CCA, Diary, October, 1918, ADM/12/5/141, NAG; Fuller, CCA, Diary, November and December, 1918, ADM/12/5/160, NAG; *Colonial Reports, Ashanti,* 1918.

40. *Colonial Reports,* Ashanti, 1918; Fuller, CCA, Diary, 10 April 1919, ADM/1624, NAG; Sir Francis Fuller, *A Vanished Dynasty: Ashanti* (London, 1921), p. 224. The estimate of 9000 deaths as 2 percent of the population would mean a population of approximately 450,000. The census in 1911 gave a figure of 287,814 for Ashanti, the census of 1921 gave 407,000, both considered low.

41. *Colonial Reports,* Ashanti, 1918.

42. The census in 1921 returned a figure of 18,085. The estimate in 1918 was 30,185, but this was one of a series of what seem to have been annual overestimates.

43. *Departmental Reports,* Report of the Medical and Sanitary Department, 1918.

44. Interview, Arnold Anderson Agbolosso, Kumasi, 22 May 1970.

45. Scott, *Epidemic Disease,* p. 100.

46. *Ibid.,* pp. 85–86.

47. Lorena, Junior Sanitary Officer to Senior Sanitary Officer, Accra, 4 March 1920, D/1255, NAG/K.

48. P. S. Selwyn-Clarke, *Report on the outbreak of plague in Kumasi, Ashanti,* Gold Coast Sessional Paper 11, 1925–26 (1926). This is a very complete report, and unless otherwise indicated the information for the plague that follows is derived from this source. The author was one of the most energetic and competent men to serve in the British colonial medical service, and is probably the only one to make a later transition to the administrative service and eventually become a colonial governor.

49. There was one case subsequently, but it could be traced to Kumasi.

50. *Departmental Reports,* Report of the Medical and Sanitary Department, 1924–25; Interview, Sir Selwyn Selwyn-Clarke, London, 12 December 1970; Interview, James Agyei Kyem, Kumasi, 18 March 1970.

51. One would have to presume that if the disease were newly introduced from Sekondi there was no epizootic prior to the first case in Kumasi, which came some two weeks after Sekondi was placed under quarantine, but the initial outbreak in Kumasi was limited.

52. Selwyn-Clarke, *Report on the outbreak;* J. Maxwell, CCA to Acting Colonial Secretary, Accra, July 1924, C/370, NAG/K.

53. Cases of primary pneumonic and septicaemic plague were invariably fatal. Case mortality for bubonic plague was 79 percent.

54. Selwyn-Clarke, *Report on the outbreak;* Minutes of the Kumasi Sanitary Committee, 10 March 1925, in the records of the Kumasi City Council.

55. J. Maxwell, CCA to Acting Colonial Secretary, Accra, 13 August 1924, C/370, NAG/K.

56. Selwyn-Clarke, *Report on the outbreak;* Interview, Arnold Anderson Agbolosoo, Kumasi, 22 May 1970.

57. Selwyn-Clarke, *Report on the outbreak;* J. Maxwell, CCA to Colonial Secretary, Accra, 29 October 1924, C/370, NAG/K; Minutes of the Kumasi Sanitary Committee, 19 June 1924, D/2385, NAG/K; J. Maxwell, CCA to Acting Colonial Secretary, Accra, July 1924, C/370, NAG/K; Interview, Sir Selwyn Selwyn-Clarke, London, 12 December 1970; Interview, I. K. Agyeman, Kumasi, 24 March 1970.

58. O. A. G. Maxwell to Colonial Secretary, London, 16 August 1924, GC 679/1924, CO/96/649, PRO.

59. Selwyn-Clarke, *Report on the outbreak; Departmental Reports,* Report of the Medical and Sanitary Department, 1924–25.

60. Minutes of the Kumasi Sanitary Committee, 13 January 1925, D/2385, NAG/K.

61. Selwyn-Clarke, *Report on the outbreak; Departmental Reports,* Report of the Medical and Sanitary Department, 1930–31.

62. Annual Reports of the Kumasi Public Health Board, 1926–27 and 1927–28; Howells, Senior Sanitary Officer, 26 April 1928, Annual Report of the Sanitary Department (Ashanti), 1927–28.

63. Annual Report of the Kumasi Public Health Board, 1927–28; Howells, Senior Sanitary Officer, 26 April 1928, Annual Report on the Sanitary Department (Ashanti), 1927–28.

64. *Departmental Reports,* Report of the Medical and Sanitary Department, 1930–31; Annual Report, Eastern Province, Ashanti, 1930–31, ADM 5/1/107, NAG.

65. Annual Report of the Kumasi Public Health Board, 1929–30.

8

Louse-Borne Relapsing Fever in Sudan, 1908–51

Gerald W. Hartwig

From 1921 until 1928 a virulent louse-borne relapsing fever epidemic moved steadily and destructively along the east/west caravan route south of the Sahara Desert. In 1921 West African troops returning from Syria may have introduced the disease when they disembarked from their ships in Conakry, Guinea, and dispersed into interior cities such as Bamako.[1] The major course of the epidemic's sporadic but steady movement is easily discernible.[2] The general direction was always eastward. Once the epidemic emerged on the Niger River, however, it moved in all directions, accompanying unsuspecting travelers wherever they went. By 1924 the epidemic was in southern Niger and still moving eastward, seemingly trapped in the grassland corridor between the desert to the north and the wetter regions to the south. In 1925 it was firmly entrenched in Chad. The epidemic remained unchecked after four years, during which a relatively few medical officials from British and French colonies worked unsuccessfully to halt its relentless progress. By mid-1926 louse-borne relapsing fever reached the western part of Sudan, in the province of Darfur. In Darfur health officials confronted, stopped, and eventually conquered the epidemic after an eighteen-month ordeal.

Between the end of the epidemic in 1928 and 1951, louse-borne relapsing fever posed a serious threat to the well-being of Sudanese. The following discussion of relapsing fever outlines the encounter between medical officials, the affected population, and the disease to illustrate three basic issues. Each issue reveals an essential correlation between health care and epidemic disease on the one hand and colonial response and responsibility on the other.

The first issue deals with the official response to an epidemic. We are partially able to discern the official attitude regarding capability, resources, and gravity of the situation through annual reports and articles in medical or general journals. Thus the methods and resources used in combatting louse-borne relapsing fever, as well as the justification for doing so, are reasonably clear. Between 1926 and 1951 the epidemiology of the disease is also easy to follow from official sources, although at an admittedly superficial level. Unfortunately the response of the people directly affected by the disease is missing from the records. A second issue deals with demographic concerns. The relapsing fever epidemics in Sudan had varying consequences for the infected population depending upon where people lived. Not only did the colonial regime indirectly promote epidemic disease through increased communication, but it also determined which of the threatened districts, and therefore which people, would receive preferential treatment. The data indicate, for example, that some regions experienced significantly and consistently higher mortality from relapsing fever than others. Such a discrepancy raises questions regarding regional differences in population growth/decline as well as administrative priorities in health and economic issues. A third issue reveals the level of medical knowledge during a particular historical period and how a major breakthrough in the production of pesticides changed relapsing fever from a serious health menace to a nuisance within a quarter of a century.

In many respects relapsing fever resembles a number of other febrile diseases, especially typhus. The initial sign of illness is a high fever, 40–40.5°C (104–105°F) or even higher. A severe headache and pain in the back, chest, abdomen, legs, and joints accompany the fever. Nausea and vomiting may also occur. Patients are apathetic, mentally dull, or simply confused. The initial attack of fever normally lasts five to seven days and then the temperature drops below normal to 36°C (96.8°F) or lower. After three or four days the fever reoccurs but for a shorter duration. If death is caused by the disease itself instead of by pneumonia or other complications, it normally occurs during the initial attack of fever. Both lice and people are necessary for the occurrence of the disease. A louse infected with the spirochete *Borrelia recurrentis* infects a person who, wittingly or unwittingly, crushes the insect and releases the spirochetes that eventually find their way through scratches in the skin into the person's bloodstream. By the same token, an infected person infects a louse which ingests the person's blood. Once the person is infected the incubation period lasts four to eight days.[3]

Relapsing fever in Sudan has gone through three distinct phases since 1900. During the initial period, from 1908 through 1925, the infection was present primarily among Egyptian troops stationed in Sudan.[4] Because the louse-borne variety of relapsing fever was endemic in Egypt at this time, it was assumed that Egyptians were responsible for these early cases, which totaled less than 200 during this sixteen-year period. The disease was relatively mild with only five recorded deaths. From such an experience Sudan health officials certainly had no cause for unusual concern. Effective treatment consisted of an intravenous injection of Novarsenobillon, an arsenic compound, during the early stages of the disease.

A European disease well understood by 1908, louse-borne relapsing fever presented no unusual problems for European medical officials in Sudan, except for the Sudanese lack of immunity. Although the spirochete of louse-borne relapsing fever had been detected in Europe as early as 1868, it was not linked to the louse until 1907.[5] Thus, in 1925 when officials unexpectedly reported six cases of relapsing fever along the Uganda border, health authorities took immediate steps to treat the patients and prevent the spread of the disease. Tick-borne relapsing fever was present in Uganda at the time (see chapter 3), so it was assumed that by burning resthouses used by infected persons the ticks would be destroyed. The assumption proved correct. The first quarter of the twentieth century ended with no recorded relapsing fever epidemic, whether louse or tick-borne, in Sudan; the few cases that had been reported were judiciously handled, thereby preventing the emergence of either epidemic or endemic conditions. Nonetheless, relapsing fever may well have been present in Sudan before 1900. It had probably existed in Egypt before 1900. And, because of the influx of Egyptians into Sudan during the nineteenth century, the possibility of an earlier introduction exists. But the absence of endemicity between 1900 and 1925 is convincing evidence that the disease in recent times had never been a serious health problem before 1926.

In August 1926 the scene altered completely. Relapsing fever suddenly became an extremely serious health hazard with economic and political effects for the Anglo-Egyptian Sudan.[6] For the next quarter of a century (with a brief respite between 1933 and 1935) the disease was an almost constant threat. From 1926 to 1932, indeed, its claim on human life was apparently too awesome for the medical service to report its magnitude.

We know little about the relapsing fever epidemic that broke out in Darfur Province in 1926. Our ignorance is a reflection of the token administrative presence in western Sudan, particularly that of the medical service. It was probably a disastrous, a murderous epidemic that decimated the population. No official estimate of cases was ever recorded, although varying numbers of deaths were given in various reports and consistently revolved around 10,000, 20,000, and 200,000: unbelievably disparate figures. Sudanese officials successfully prevented the epidemic from moving eastward into the province of Kordofan when the epidemic was in its most virulent stage, a remarkable feat under the existing conditions.

Although the Sudan medical staff may have been physically isolated from the medical staffs of other African colonies, we should be able to assume some communication between the various colonial administrations, even if one (Chad) was administered by the French and the other (Sudan) by the British. But the available evidence reveals a state of ignorance on the part of the Sudan Medical Service that is difficult to explain.

In early 1926 G. K. Maurice was posted as Senior Medical Officer in Darfur Province. From his general description of the epidemic and his role in combatting it we have some knowledge

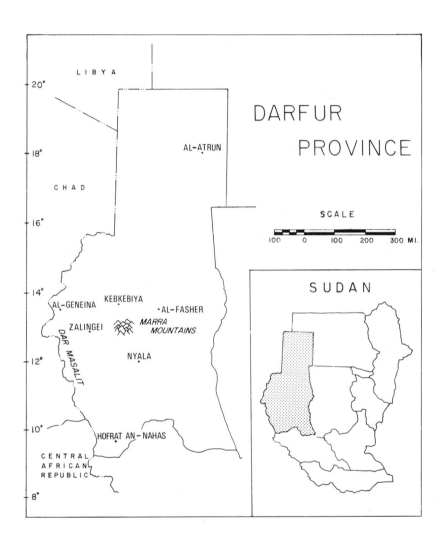

of conditions surrounding the epidemic.[7] Maurice was stationed at the provincial administrative center at El Fasher in the eastern part of Darfur. His trained staff consisted of three Syrian medical officers: one posted at El Fasher, one at Nyala, and the third at Geneina, a town situated on the major east/west route on the Chad border. The medical staff also included a total of four military *tumergis* or Dispensary Hakims, two stationed at Kebkebia and two at Zalingei. A *tumergi* had a rudimentary medical training enabling him to qualify as a medical dispenser. These eight men had responsibility for the health care of some 750,000 people in Darfur, a huge province of 138,150 square miles. In 1926 a few rudimentary roads existed in Darfur, but automobiles were scarce and only available to the Medical Service on an emergency basis. Virtually all travel was by camel. Desert was the norm in the northern part of the province, inhabited by nomadic Arabs. Inaccessible mountains, inhabited by an agricultural population, characterized the center of the province. Furthermore, the administration had been present in Darfur for only ten years, and was more a military than a civil regime. Not surprisingly, "the average Fur [a major agricultural ethnic group in Darfur] looked on the medical authorities and their works with profound suspicion."[8] Another medical officer referred to the "fatalistic character of the inhabitants," reinforcing the impression that their cooperation during the epidemic was minimal at best.[9]

Maurice first heard of a potential health problem on 26 June 1926, but the affected population denied the existence of any sickness. The information was consequently treated as a rumor. In August health officials in Khartoum sent a routine report warning that relapsing fever was present in the easternmost Chadian province of Wadai. Maurice warned the Syrian medical officer at the border town of Geneina to watch for possible carriers of the disease entering Sudan from Wadai. He also requested that specimens of lice, bed bugs, and particularly ticks be brought to him for transmission to the Wellcome Tropical Research Laboratories in Khartoum to determine which insect was the vector. He later wrote: "Looking back now [1932] it seems to be obvious that I should have suspected first of all the louse. However I knew

nothing at this time of the disease having spread across Africa."[10]
Knowing which vector was involved, the louse or the tick, would
naturally determine how to combat the disease. Ignorant of the
louse-borne relapsing fever epidemic that has been approaching
from the west since 1921, Maurice suspected the tick. His previous experience had been in the southern province of Equatoria
(then called Bahr al Ghazal) where he had campaigned against
sleeping sickness for four years. His general knowledge of relapsing fever was limited to the six reported cases of tick-borne relapsing fever in 1925 in Equatoria Province that had occurred
just before he was posted to Darfur Province.

Maurice's ignorance can be understood: he was a medical officer in the field, dependent upon others for knowledge of developments outside his assigned area. Ignorance or a lack of concern
among health officials in Khartoum is another matter. Relapsing
fever had been reported from colonies to the west since 1921.
The gradual movement eastward should have been apparent.
Descriptions of the epidemic had appeared by 1925 in medical
journals and in reports from the Health Section of the League of
Nations. Although several articles were in French publications,[11]
a discussion of the epidemic in northern Nigeria was published
in London in the *Journal of Tropical Medicine and Hygiene,* in
which it was reported that an estimated 128,750 people had died
in Kano Province alone.[12] Either through the reading of such
professional journals or through the communication of relevant
officials in London, the Sudan Medical Service should have been
aware of the possible spread of the epidemic into Sudan. Apparently they were not. Even medical officials in Chad did not
inform Sudan officials until October 1926 about the dangers of
the epidemic, some 21 months after it has been detected in Chad.
While cooperation between Chadian and Sudanese officials was
officially announced on 25 October 1926, the action to curtail
travel and thus the spread of the epidemic occurred too late to
prevent its progress into Darfur Province.[13] How the Sudan Medical Service initially learned of the epidemic in Chad was not
made clear in the annual report.[14] It simply refers to the local
outbreaks in September, describes the epidemic's presence in

Africa since 1921, and mentions that the knowledge of the louse as vector was never really in doubt, thereby glossing over a number of very serious problems:

Cases of relapsing fever were reported from the Kebkebia district on September 11, 1926 and a similar outbreak was reported from the Nyala district on September 12. It became clear that the whole of the northern Zalingei area was heavily infected and that in addition serious outbreaks, with a very heavy case mortality estimated at 60–80%, were present in the Kebkebia and Nyala districts.

Since louse-borne relapsing fever had been epidemic in West Africa since 1921 and more recently had spread to the Tchad region and to Wadai it was decided to treat this disease as being louse-borne pending further investigation.[15]

If health officials in Khartoum had so much knowledge about the nature of the relapsing fever epidemic in Chad, it was inexcusable not to have passed such information on to Maurice. Nevertheless, the Sudan Medical Service was late in learning about the epidemic in Chad and originally had no idea whether the tick or the louse was the vector. On 20 October Maurice declared that "Khartoum was worrying me at this time for a definite answer as to whether the disease was louse, or tick borne. I was still puzzled but the louse was more and more suspected."[16] A month earlier, on 20 September, Maurice had confirmed that the disease was, as suspected, relapsing fever. Having requested a large supply of Novarsenobillon and syringes, he could fight the epidemic, albeit in a sledge-hammer fashion: he had to contend with both ticks and lice. Since ticks infested buildings, officials burned all living quarters in infected villages.[17] Not until 7 December did the Wellcome Research Laboratories confirm the louse as the responsible vector.[18] All efforts then focused upon delousing inhabitants of infected regions. Thus the official report of the Medical Service avoided the discussion of two embarrassing issues: why knowledge of the five-year old epidemic was so long in reaching Khartoum and why the vector responsible for the epidemic should have posed such a problem for so long.

Once the seriousness of the epidemic was apparent, the Medical Service and other administrative officials in Darfur acted commendably. The disease was acute, with mortality soaring to some 70 percent of its victims. The motivation of officials no doubt varied, but within official reports the justification for the impressive effort and expense is clear: "The question arises, will it be possible to check this disease on the eastern borders of Darfur or will it inevitably spread through Kordofan to the thickly populated area of the Gezirah [*sic*]."[19] Checking the spread of relapsing fever became the official goal: "A disease of high virulence attacking the non-immune and lice-ridden dense population of the Gezira on the same scale as it attacked Darfur, would have been a social and economic disaster."[20] Dr. Robert Kirk succinctly expressed the economic goal a decade after the initial epidemic was stopped: "Had it invaded Gezira, the work in the cotton-fields would have been seriously disorganized, and the whole Sudan might have been faced with an economic disaster of the first magnitude."[21] In 1934 Harold MacMichael, a respected former Civil Secretary of Sudan, also gave an economic justification: "it was urgently necessary to wage war upon the numerous endemic and epidemic diseases which were restricting the growth of the population and lowering its standard of productivity. . . . In 1925 and 1926 two diseases in particular gave cause for serious alarm. The first was *bilharzia*. . . . The second, and more deadly, menace was relapsing fever. . . ."[22] The Anglo-Egyptian Sudan had a very limited economic base. Virtually all resources were marshaled for implementing a cotton growing project in the Gezira area along the Blue Nile. In 1925 the project showed the first signs of success. Hence the relapsing fever epidemic in late 1926 was a development that threatened the lifeline of the colony. The threat was met with "a heavy expenditure of energy and money. . . . It was controlled before it spread into Kordofan at a cost of at least £E. 40,000 and 20,000 lives."[23]

The Sudan Medical Service did not keep systematic statistics until 1930. Its reluctant estimation of cases and mortality was based on two figures that repeatedly occur in various contexts. The estimate of 20,000 appears significantly understated. But one factor is constant in the literature: the cost in lives was very high, and therefore alarming to the administration. The *Annual*

Report for 1926 gives one estimate: "The mortality in Zalingei district had been very heavy. The deaths in this area were estimated at 10,000 out of a total population of 45,000."[24] The source of this estimate was probably Dr. D. Riding, Assistant Bacteriologist at the Wellcome Tropical Research Laboratories in Khartoum, and Dr. T. W. MacDowell, Medical Inspector, Sudan Medical Service. They estimated that there had been 10,000 deaths in the Zalingei area but gave the total population as 40,000 rather than 45,000.[25] On the other hand, Maurice, the Senior Medical Officer in Darfur, noted that there had been "six thousand deaths in Zalingei District" during the last six months of 1926.[26] The number 6,000 was never subsequently used in official or unofficial reports. In his article in *Sudan Notes and Records*, Maurice used the figure 10,000 to estimate relapsing fever deaths in Darfur, instead of simply the Zalingei district: "In 1926 relapsing fever killed ten thousand of the population of Darfur in the space of six months."[27] The *Annual Report for 1926* retained the figure of 10,000 while restricting it to one of five districts, suggesting a higher toll for the entire province. Subsequent annual reports studiously avoided estimating cases of the disease or deaths caused by it. Not until 1933 was there an official composite figure of 20,000 for total mortality.[28] Because the epidemic was concentrated in one province and the efforts to contain it were given such high priority, it is difficult to understand why the Medical Service avoided recording the estimated mortality from the disease until 1933. Even when the estimated total of 20,000 deaths appeared, it was so low that it is necessary to question the figure and to suspect that there was a reason for such a small number.

The evidence indicates a significantly higher mortality. Probably the best informed man was Maurice. Apart from the figures of 6,000 he gave for Zalingei District and 10,000 for the province as a whole, he avoided specifics, except on a local basis. For example, he mentioned visiting eleven infected villages, with 60 relapsing fever patients; those eleven villages had already experienced 153 deaths from the disease.[29] In two other instances he resorted to estimated proportions of the population. Such a device is useful if the total population is known; unfortunately he did not provide that information. But the devastation of the epidemic is all too clear: "I had found that the disease commonly swept through a village and infected a half or a third of the population, with a case mortality of about 70%, after which its virulence abated."[30] In his conclusion Maurice compared the effect of the epidemic in Darfur, where it "killed nearly a quarter of the Fur population of the Sudan," to the Black Death in England which, he claimed, killed half of the English population in 1488.[31]

Estimates of the population of Darfur vary. If we examine the first population census taken in 1955–56, the total population of Darfur Province was given as 902,798; the Fur alone numbered 303,173, or about one-third of the total.[32] The percentage of Fur in relation to the total population of Darfur has probably not altered substantially during the twentieth century, unless the relapsing fever epidemic afflicted the Fur to an extraordinary degree while causing much less mortality among non-Fur. There is no data to support such a possibility. Thus when Maurice referred to the Fur losing about one-fourth of their numbers, this in addition to losses from neighboring non-Fur, the estimate of 20,000 deaths becomes strangely inadequate. But there is additional conflicting information. In 1926 a Medical Service report to the League of Nations estimated the population of Darfur at 750,000;[33] in 1929 the official smallpox report of the Medical Service gave the population of Darfur as 500,000.[34] The estimated population for the province by the same government agency decreased without explanation by 250,000 in three years.

Two other pieces of evidence question the official mortality reports. The systematic reporting of statistics by the Medical Service was not fully inaugurated until 1930. Yet in the reports of 1928 and 1929 we find the Medical Service giving precise information from Darfur Province on the number of reported cases and deaths from a smallpox epidemic that erupted as the relapsing fever epidemic was waning.[35] Although the staff and mechanism for reporting and recording medical data were available in Darfur by the first part of 1927, statistics for relapsing fever do

not appear until 1930. The second piece of evidence comes from
C. E. G. Beveridge, an official in the Sudan Medical Service. He
published a brief report in January 1928, when the epidemic was
under control but still in existence. His introductory paragraph
is worth citing for the surprisingly high mortality asserted, presumably for Darfur, and for the matter-of-fact manner in which
the entire epidemic is treated:

> The probable origin of relapsing fever in Africa was from the black
> troops returning to French West Africa after the war in 1921. It has
> spread over British and French West Africa, reaching Wadai in 1926
> and thence into Darfur, the most western province of the Anglo-
> Egyptian Sudan. The mortality has reached epidemic figures. Reports
> as to the number of deaths must of necessity be somewhat inaccurate;
> however, a total of 200,000 deaths is probably a low estimate.[36]

In addition to the figure of 200,000, two other factors are of
interest: the article was written before the epidemic was over
and, presumably, before the *Annual Report for 1927;* also, the
article was "published with the kind permission of O. F. H.
Atkey, Esq., F. R. C. S., Director of the Sudan Medical Service."[37]
Thus it seems that in early 1927 the most senior official in the
Medical Service was not apparently concerned about publishing
high estimates of mortality. But shortly thereafter estimates
ceased appearing until the 20,000 composite figure of 1933, a
figure that is grossly understated if Beveridge and Maurice are
to be believed.

A controversy regarding the introduction of relapsing fever
emerged among those writing about the epidemic. With good
reason, health officials in Sudan assumed that outsiders were responsible for most problems. The standard explanation implicated "travellers, especially pilgrims, to Mecca, as numbers pass
through Darfur every year from West Africa."[38] Kirk added another dimension to the explanation: "The epidemiology of relapsing fever in the Sudan during the last twelve years has been
very largely determined by the habits and movements of [west-
erners]." They frequently traveled, according to Kirk, in search
of temporary work. Some, once they possessed enough money to
buy cattle, returned to their own country. Others participated

each November and December in the cotton harvest in Gezira, and continued on their pilgrimage to Mecca.[39]

Kirk assumed that travelers from Chad, or persons passing through Chad from further west, entered Sudan during August or September of 1926 and thus spread the epidemic.[40] He rejected the possibility suggested by Riding and MacDowell that there was a "small endemic area of relapsing fever" in the Marra Mountains, situated in the center of Darfur.[41] But unlike anyone else in Darfur, Riding and MacDowell had made enquiries about the disease and had heard that something similar to it had existed for four years in the Marra Mountains. The two men did not go to the Marra Mountains to pursue their questioning, but they confidently asserted that travelers had not recently introduced the disease. They gave three significant reasons to support their contention that pilgrims (Fellata) had not introduced the disease, at least recently: they had observed no case of relapsing fever among the Fellata, who normally did not socialize with inhabitants of districts through which they passed anyway; Dar Masalit, a district 25 to 40 miles wide between French territory and Darfur, was practically uninfected; and no cases occurred in Geneina, the border town situated on the main east/west route. The cases were concentrated to the southeast of Geneina on the road to Zalingei.[42] Although Riding and MacDowell made these observations during November and December 1926, two to three months after the initial reports warned of an epidemic, it is doubtful that their information would have been totally incorrect. It is more likely that they had stumbled onto a significant factor related to the time of introduction.

The assumption that relapsing fever was endemic in the Marra Mountains of Darfur resolved their difficulty in finding evidence to support the thesis that the epidemic was recently introduced from Chad. The fact that the border town of Geneina reported no stricken pilgrims nor any other cases could be understood only if the disease were already established in Darfur before September 1926. It was also evident that the epidemic involved local inhabitants, not travelers.[43] The incidence of the disease among the sexes confirms this. Riding and MacDowell examined

53 male patients and 47 female patients;[44] Beveridge reported on 116 patients, of whom 59 were female and 57 were male.[45] When travelers, whether pilgrims or laborers, were involved there was no sex balance among the patients because women seldom traveled for these reasons. The percentage of male patients was consistently over 90 percent.[46] The near-equal incidence in both sexes suggests that the disease had been present in Darfur before the initial cases were reported. Maurice's rumor of trouble in June was no doubt close to correct. How close is difficult to ascertain. Wadai in neighboring Chad had reported its first cases in December 1924, eighteen months before.[47] The disease could easily have been introduced in Darfur any time during the latter part of 1925 or the first half of 1926, giving Riding and MacDowell the impression of endemicity.

The controversy revolving around endemicity did not determine how or when the disease was actually introduced. Riding and MacDowell did not resolve the inconsistencies they had uncovered, and the always available westerner or pilgrim was assigned the dubious honor of introducing the epidemic into Darfur. The truth of the matter remains unknown, like so many other features of this awesome epidemic. But it was certainly a more complex process than the reports revealed.

During the latter part of 1926 and all of 1927, the role assumed by the Sudan Medical Service in combatting the epidemic was impressive given limited staff and difficult conditions. The following discussion of this phase of the epidemic has no controversy to report, nothing embarrassing that was quietly neglected in reports and henceforth officially forgotten. Furthermore social and economic motives for preventing the spread of the epidemic were readily accepted by all concerned parties. The entire administration had a stake in the outcome of the struggle.

According to the official report, written during the height of the epidemic, the administration was doing all in its power to stop the potential disaster. Within the infected areas, Maurice and his staff isolated the sick in temporary shelters and treated them with Novarsenobillon. All infected villages, as well as contiguous villages, were systematically deloused, a process that continued for three to six weeks after the last reported case. During the delousing the villages had to be temporarily evacuated. Especially dirty villages were moved to new sites more accessible to the rudimentary road system. The administration also tried as far as possible to prevent people from moving from infected to noninfected areas.[48]

The official report insisted that, from the start, the louse had been known to be the vector. But initially Maurice and his staff fought both the louse and the tick. They concentrated on a few villages with a high rate of infection, where they deloused the uninfected population and burned all dwellings in the village. The inhabitants of Darfur generally "regarded being deloused as rather a joke, but do not like it," Maurice conceded.[49] Delousing normally involved ridding the head and the clothing of lice. Men had their heads shaved whereas women had a mixture of fat and kerosene put into their hair to kill the lice. Clothing was boiled for one minute and then returned to the owner. When cases of relapsing fever continued to occur in rebuilt villages, Maurice realized (before laboratory tests confirmed it) that the louse was the responsible vector. Thus the policy of burning villages to destroy ticks could stop. But they learned from experience that clothing had to be boiled for ten consecutive days to free a village from lice. Such measures as delousing and burning provoked resistance from the victims. Typical of the misunderstanding that frequently characterized the relationship between the colonizer and the colonized, Maurice described the Fur as difficult to work with. They concealed their sick, hid their clothing, pulled down the isolation booths which were used for disrobing, and received visitors from infected villages.[50]

Preventing the epidemic's movement eastward from village to village was an immense problem for four doctors and four dispensers in the huge province. Controlling the main routes was much easier. Sick travelers were detained, and delousing stations were set up to prevent the epidemic's spread into the province of Kordofan. Had such a procedure been followed earlier at the Chadian border, the fight against the epidemic could have started before the devastation ever reached Darfur. Maurice assumed he could control the movement of people along the major routes, but those who did not use major routes concerned him: "The danger, I feared, was a gradual spread eastward village by village, rather than infection of Kordofan or the Gezira by pilgrims and travelers."[51] In late 1926 he realized that a much larger staff was urgently needed. If such reinforcements were not made available, Maurice planned to locate all available personnel on the eastern edge of Darfur Province and thereby stop the movement of people, simultaneously "leaving infected areas to their own fate."[52] Such a retreat could have horrible consequences: "News had already reached us from French territory [Chad] that the cattle there were wandering unattended, so few were the survivors of the epidemic."[53] On 17 December Maurice sent a telegram to Khartoum reflecting the desperate situation.

Relapsing fever situation [is] very serious and cannot be controlled without great increase [of] staff, approximately 12 medical officers and 30 tumergis. . . . Have definitely established fact that disease can be stamped out in limited areas sufficiently supervised. Estimate one year sufficient [to] arrest epidemic if staff [is] available. Eastern spread temporarily controlled but fear [we] cannot continue so indefinitely with big reservoir [of disease] in Zalingei.[54]

Maurice's superiors immediately sent additional help to Darfur. A serious commitment was made to combat the epidemic in December 1926, regardless of overwhelming odds against success. Major difficulties included the difficulty and length of time required to transport staff and supplies from the railhead at El Obeid in Kordofan Province to El Fasher in Darfur; the indigenous population who were likely to disappear into the mountains when health officials appeared; the inaccessibility of mountain villages where the disease was deeply entrenched; the lack of roads in the province; and drought in some parts of Darfur which meant that grain and pasture were available only in the highly infected Marra Mountains. Administrators outside the Medical Service also recognized the serious threat and cooperated in all quarantine measures and in the immediate improvement of roads and communications. The official report for 1926, however, was not optimistic; the obstacles seemed beyond the capabilities of the meager staff.[55]

By late December Maurice had developed and subsequently implemented his plan for the establishment of ten medical units. Each unit was to be led by a physician with ten *tumergis* under his supervision. Because training was necessary to become a *tumergi* and because existing *tumergi* were so few in number, Maurice had to locate prospective candidates on the streets of El Fasher. The candidates were then instructed in the twin arts of delousing and giving injections. By mid-March of 1927 Maurice could see that progress was being made. The key to success was a quick response to any reported outbreak. If a medical unit could get to a newly infected area rapidly, the disease could be controlled and the victims cured. The use of automobiles reduced the time required to reach afflicted areas. More importantly, local headmen began to request medical assistance as soon as possible rather than attempting to hide the fact.[56] Although the indignities associated with delousing remained, the benefits of the injections assumed greater importance. For those receiving injections, mortality was about 7 percent, mostly among persons weakened by prolonged illness. Among those not receiving injections of Novarsenobillon, mortality approximated 70 percent.[57]

Relapsing fever was extremely virulent in Darfur, but not everyone was affected in the same manner. One reaction was "acute fulminating"; death was typically within 48 hours, during the period of high fever. These victims seldom lived long enough to receive an injection. A second type was "ordinary severe." Among these cases there was also heavy mortality, unless an injection was received. Convalescence in survivors was prolonged and many deaths were caused by respiratory complications. The third type was "mild ambulatory" and was common during the epidemic. During the later stages of this type of infection, the patient showed signs of anemia, but never felt severely ill. These people posed the greatest problem in controlling the epidemic because they continued to spread the disease by traveling from one village to another.[58]

By late 1927 the epidemic was controlled. It was then a matter of responding to sporadic outbreaks. Delousing operations and rigid quarantines were discontinued. The Medical Service had gained confidence in its operation and enough of the inhabitants of Darfur had acquired confidence in the Medical Service for relapsing fever to be viewed as a manageable disease. The entire system, however, depended upon prompt information, and promptness depended upon cooperation. To encourage promptness in reporting outbreaks, "delousing operations are reduced to a minimum where early information of an outbreak is given and the supplier of information is rewarded with money."[59] Future efforts against epidemics in Darfur revolved around the establishment after 1927 of fourteen small dispensaries scattered throughout the province. Such units would provide knowledge about local conditions and the staff to meet emergencies, while improved communication and transportation would enable all available resources to be used against local problems before they mushroomed into regional problems.[60] It is interesting to see so much emphasis placed upon knowledge (intelligence) in this particular report since it was the lack of it that had led to the devastating consequences of the epidemic and the apparent attempt by the administration to minimize the loss of life in its reports.

The abolition of delousing stations in late 1927, before the disease had been completely eradicated, appears almost foolhardy given the administration's urgency and fear only a year earlier. But the Medical Service's newly acquired confidence in handling relapsing fever was greatly facilitated by the altering nature of the disease itself. The acutely virulent form seemed to have burned itself out in Darfur; it very seldom caused death during the initial days of fever as the former acute fulminating type had. During 1928 and 1929 the epidemic showed signs of dying out. Then in 1930, just as relapsing fever statistics became available for the first time, the disease appeared in the Gezira. But relapsing fever was now controllable. The economically sensitive province of Blue Nile, in which Gezira was located, reported 386 cases of whom 46 persons died. As was expected, westerners accounted for 98.2 percent of these cases.[61] By 1933, not a single case of relapsing fever was reported in the entire country. The second phase of relapsing fever in Sudan was over. In summarizing its effort to control the epidemic, the Medical Service mentioned the cost in money (£E. 40,000) and lives (20,000). The specter of what might have happened was also reiterated.

The disease was never a factor of any importance in the important central provinces but there would have been a very different tale to tell if the efforts to prevent its spread eastwards in 1926 had not been successful. A disease of high virulence attacking the non-immune and lice ridden dense population of the Gezira on the same scale as it attacked Darfur, would have been a social and economic disaster.[62]

The interlude between the second and third phases of relapsing fever in Sudan was a brief but no doubt welcome reprieve for all concerned with delousing. Only one isolated case of the disease was reported between 1933 and 1935. In 1936, 22 cases signaled the onset of another strenuous bout with the disease, a protracted struggle that for all practical purposes took fifteen years to complete.

The 22 cases without mortality during 1936 became 374 the following year but accompanied by a mortality of 12.8 percent (48 deaths), a figure similar to that recorded in 1930 (11.9 percent) and 1931 (13.4 percent). The official report for 1937 noted that the disease was largely confined to and spread by West African immigrants. Fortunately it was not a particularly virulent strain; early treatment normally cured the patient. With the usual precautions it was presumed possible to keep the disease under control and to avoid a heavy general infection of a high mortality. During 1937, a total of 25,381 persons passed through delousing stations.[63] The report of that year was cautiously couched in optimistic terms.

As with the outbreak of relapsing fever in 1926, responsibility for this later one was attributed to outsiders, only this time the outsiders came from Ethiopia (Abyssinia) and Eritrea. Unlike the epidemic of 1926, however, there was an adequate investigation. Robert Kirk studied the situation in 1936 and 1937 to determine the reasons for the appearance of migrants in Sudan and where they might have encountered the disease. The emergence of relapsing fever in 1936 was indirectly linked to the Italian invasion of Ethiopia in 1935; however, it was not brought in by Ethiopian refugees, but by the ubiquitous westerner again. According to Kirk, after the military occupation by the Italians, there was a general assumption that the invaders would require labor. Therefore "a large migration of Westerners had been deflected into Eritrea and Abyssinia during the previous two years, in the reasonable expectation that they would there find a market where labour would command high prices."[64] But the conditions there had been disappointing. Labor had been needed, primarily for road building, but frequently under very difficult conditions. The available food and the climate were unpleasantly different as well; disease, both smallpox and a type of fever, took its toll. Those who had earned and saved money found that they could not take it out of the country because of currency restrictions. Disillusioned, portions of this mobile labor population began returning to Sudan in 1936. A few of them introduced relapsing fever.

The victims and carriers of the disease during the late 1930s were a remarkably homogeneous group because the disease was originally identified with migrant laborers in the Blue Nile Province. The affected population was then predominantly male and western in origin. Kirk likened these immigrants to refugees: they had neither water for washing nor satisfactory living accommodations. They were dirty, tired, harassed, and ill-fed, and they and their clothing provided an excellent environment for lice.[65]

Despite the optimism of 1937, the Medical Service found itself battling a persistent disease in 1938. The 374 cases in 1937[66] grew to 1,124 cases in 1938, leading to the latter year's pessimistic report.[67] By 1938 the irrigated cotton country in the Gezira had 670 reported cases, although the disease remained under control. Only 51 patients died, a mortality of 7.6 percent. The major concern of the Medical Service was Darfur where the epidemic might "rage out of control again."[68] The dispensaries simply could not serve the dispersed population adequately. Consequently, of the 212 reported cases in Darfur, there were 45 deaths, a mortality of 21 percent.[69] Dr. Kirk explicitly acknowledged the problem of health services in Darfur. During 1937, the average mortality for all cases in Sudan was some 12 percent, but this average masks regional differences. The mortality for Blue Nile Province was 6.2 percent (191 cases, 12 deaths) whereas for Darfur mortality was 35.3 percent.[70] Kirk feared that the comparative mortality figures from the various provinces indicated the seriousness of the disease, even when the acute fulminating form was absent. Darfur's statistics, reflecting fewer medical facilities and therefore a lower standard of health care, revealed the potential danger: "Probably, therefore, the Darfur mortality is much nearer what the figure for the untreated disease would be, and suggests that in the absence of proper medical and sanitary measures this disease might very well repeat the havoc of former years."[71] Furthermore, the staff of the Medical Service conceded that it was "impossible to prevent the spread of the disease" because it was carried by a "shy, wandering, foreign population which wends its way casually across the Sudan to and from Mecca."[72] Sick persons could be easily stopped and quarantined, but carriers of the disease who were not ill enough to be noticed continued to infect and reinfect strategic sites along their route. Efforts to eradicate the disease in the late 1930s did not meet the success of the early 1930s.

As shown in Table 1, the total number of cases declined slightly in 1939. The Medical Service deloused some 100,000 persons in that year, four times the number deloused two years earlier.[73] In 1940 the number of cases approached 1,500. The officials laconically declared that the "disease now appears to be endemic in Sudan." Henceforth it would be necessary to practice rigorous preventive measures.[74] The reported cases during 1941 continued their upward climb. The average mortality of 3.6 percent, however, suggests an improvement in health care. But such a conclusion is premature. Because only four cases of relapsing fever occurred in Darfur, the mortality average was significantly lowered. The following year, 1942, witnessed another serious outbreak in Darfur, and the average mortality increased to 10.5 per-

Table 1. *Reported Cases, Deaths, and Mortality from Louse-Borne Relapsing Fever, 1935–42*

Province	1935	1936	1937	1938	1939	1940	1941	1942
Blue Nile	0	22	191/12[a]	670/51	402/29	782/22	2954/103	3594/119
Darfur	0	0	68/24	212/45	278/46	116/9	4/1	1350/412
Kassala	0	0	95/10	158/14	117/6	551/13	9/1	50/4
Khartoum	0	0	3/1	16/0	116/3	27/0	27/2	63/1
Kordofan	0	0	16/1	66/6	72/8	11/1	29/3	194/20
Upper Nile	0	0	0	0	0	0	1/0	0
Other	0	0	1/0	2/0	21/0	0	4/0	36/3
Total Cases	0	22	374	1124	1006	1487	3024	5287
Deaths	0	0	48	116	92	45	110	559
Mortality	0	0	12.8%	10.3%	9.1%	3.0%	3.6%	10.5%

a. The first figure represents the number of cases and the second figure represents the number of deaths.
Source: Based upon the *Annual Reports* for 1935 to 1942, Sudan, Ministry of Health.

cent. Of the 1,350 cases in Darfur, the mortality was 30.5 percent (412 deaths) whereas in the Blue Nile Province the mortality was 3.3 percent (119 deaths) among 3,594 patients. These statistics reflect the varying health care facilities.

Table 2 illustrates the tremendous growth of relapsing fever during 1943 and 1944, and a sizable decrease in 1945; then the figures suddenly plummeted in 1946. Because mortality remained low during these years (even Darfur's figures remained under 20 percent), the Medical Service could take some credit for its effort. Getting the disease under control was another matter. Nonetheless, at the end of the worst year since 1930 for the number of cases of relapsing fever, the anticipated victory over the disease was mentioned in a hopeful, confident way.

The disease has been a cause of worry and of an enormous amount of additional work by the public health and dispensary staff during the war, but it is hoped that as soon as DDT powder is available it will be possible to deal with it more effectively and easily than at present.[75]

The availability of the insecticide DDT enabled the Medical Service to combat lice more effectively in 1945. Special attention was paid to the Blue Nile Province, and the cases of relapsing fever declined impressively between 1944 (14,231) and 1945 (4,698). But in 1945 the disease erupted in an epidemic in the Upper Nile Province. This province, located south of Khartoum and embracing the White Nile, was inhabited by Nilotic-speaking agriculturalists such as the Shilluk. The east/west route used by immigrants passed north of the province; therefore it did not share the same epidemiological environment as Darfur or Blue Nile Provinces. The disease was apparently introduced by Shilluk who had participated in migrant labor activities to the north and returned home with the disease. For people like the Shilluk, relapsing fever represented an index of acceptance of external modes and customs. Like many southern Sudanese early in the twentieth century, the Shilluk had a disdain for clothing. The presence of relapsing fever suggests that clothing, a haven for lice, was common among them by the mid-1940s. Nonetheless DDT solved the problem for the Shilluk as readily as it had for

Table 2. Reported Cases, Deaths, and Mortality from Louse-Borne Relapsing Fever, 1943–51

Province	1943	1944	1945	1946	1947	1948	1949	1950/51
Blue Nile	7691/226[a]	14231/68	4698/37	462/12	28/0	68/1		
Darfur	807/312	1055/109	1068/160	278/43	294/58	50/1		
Kassala	454/32	841/44	1779/58	32/2	0	19/6		
Khartoum	551/5	1878/30	681/17	4/0	0	24/0		
Kordofan	902/89	3616/21	1683/15	314/1	38/3	31/0		
Upper Nile	9/0	977/38	7474/157	840/6	228/3	87/0		
Other	91/4	74/0	9/0	22/1	?/3	8/0		
Total Cases	10,505	22,672	17,392	1952	588	287	376	36
Deaths	668	310	444	65	67	8	3	2
Mortality	6.3%	1.3%	2.5%	3.3%	11.3%	2.7%	.7%	5.5%

a. The first figure represents the number of cases and the second figure represents the number of deaths.
Source: Based upon the Annual Reports for 1943 to 1950–51, Sudan, Ministry of Health.

people in the Gezira.[76] By 1949 only 376 cases were reported in all of Sudan; the following year the figure had dropped to 36. The third phase of relapsing fever in Sudan was over. Henceforth relapsing fever lost its awesome threat to the health of Sudanese; the weapons for use against the disease and its vector were now readily available.

The response of the Sudan Medical Service to relapsing fever during the first half of the twentieth century raises three general issues: the methods and resources available to a colonial regime in Africa for use in treating a serious health problem, and the justification for doing so; the demographic consequences of serious diseases; and the impact that medical and scientific advancements had upon the colonial health care system. Although we are unable to examine the perceptions and responses of the affected Sudanese population from European sources, it is clear that methods of treating health problems (e.g., delousing and burning dwellings) caused resentment as well as resistance. That people in one province received better medical attention than those living in another also raises awkward questions.

What we have learned about methods and resources for combatting relapsing fever is not surprising. The tenacious louse is a difficult opponent, particularly among a migrating population with very little access to water and cleanliness. The procedures involved in delousing—the boiling of clothing and shaving of men's heads—were sufficiently irksome and cumbersome to insure that success would remain elusive until an effective pesticide was developed. The louse, it should be made clear, was an indigenous insect in central Sudan wherever the epidemic of 1921 to 1928 occurred. However, in this region before 1921 neither lice nor men harbored the spirochete (*Borrelia recurrentis*) responsible for relapsing fever. Because a readily available arsenical compound was known to cure the disease, control was a matter of trained personnel carrying out delousing operations and giving patients injections of Novarsenobillon. This was initially done in 1927 during the height of the epidemic in Darfur by using unskilled men from the provincial capital of El Fasher. When the Medical Service established a few widely scattered dispensaries, the standard of training necessary for the post was, presumably, increased. The one lasting benefit for the people of Darfur as a consequence of the epidemic of 1926–28 was an initiation "into modern medicine," according to Maurice. "It taught them to recognize one benefit from Government. . . . Medicine counsels peace."[77]

The economic justification for expending substantial sums of money and for sending medical personnel and provisions in 1926 to halt the spread of the epidemic from Darfur into the cotton-growing district of Gezira is understandable. But the absence of expressed humanitarian concern is striking. The silence was no doubt related to the reluctance of the people of Darfur to accept delousing and the burning of villages. By not appreciating the sincere but disruptive initial efforts of the Medical Service, they earned a reputation for being ungrateful and ignorant. Although they gradually accepted the attempts of the Medical Service, there is little indication that the European doctors made as much progress in understanding the responses of the people of Darfur.

The Medical Service's apparent desire to report a questionably low mortality estimate is one of the unforeseen results of this study. The only conceivable reason for minimizing the effect of the epidemic was to conceal the failure on the part of authorities in Khartoum and London to alert officials in Darfur that an epidemic was in progress further west and was approaching the Anglo-Egyptian Sudan. Such a lack of communication between officials from various African colonies is surprising in 1926, especially when the loss of life from the epidemic before 1926 was so high. If the absence of advanced knowledge about the epidemic ever seriously concerned Sudanese officials, there is no evidence of it in the annual reports or in related publications that discussed the epidemic. The failure of the Medical Services to refute high estimates—ranging from an inferred 125,000 to a stated 200,000—published by medical officials is disturbing, especially if it was felt that the estimates were unreasonable. Obviously other sources would have to be sought to ascertain the numerical dimensions of the epidemic and thus its impact upon the people of Darfur. Only after 1930 were statistical medical records systematically kept. Before 1930 in Anglo-Egyptian Sudan, it is apparent that medical records are incomplete and those that exist have been influenced by a desire to avoid specifics.

The demographic issues raised in this discussion are less complex. The loss of life and the illness related to louse-borne relapsing fever are very much a product of an increasingly interrelated world community. The return of West Africans to Guinea following their service in the French military and the subsequent eruption of louse-borne relapsing fever into the Sahel region of sub-Saharan Africa reflect increased communication among Africans and non-Africans. The disease affected only portions of a country like Sudan; the extreme north and south escaped the disease for ecological reasons. But even in the central region where the disease flourished, its impact differed. In the economically vital Blue Nile Province, mortality was consistently low. The low mortality was directly related to available and sufficient medical dispensaries. Conversely, the consistently higher mortality among victims of relapsing fever in Darfur Province was directly related to fewer dispensaries. From 1936 to 1948, the records indicate that Darfur Province had 5,580 cases of relapsing fever with 1,220 deaths (mortality of 21.8 percent) whereas Blue Nile Province had 35,771 cases with only 680 deaths (mortality of 1.9 percent). Thus when examining demographic variables, it is absolutely necessary to consider regional variations. A province like Darfur was marginal to the major economic endeavors of the colonial regime and its marginal status was reflected in the colonial investment in dispensaries.

On a more positive note, it is impressive to see the impact that the development and use of a pesticide like DDT could have on louse-borne relapsing fever. Equally important to note in the case of relapsing fever was the availability of a drug during the 1920s to treat and cure victims of the disease. Thus the disease could be controlled if the specific medicine and trained people were available. By the same token, a high death toll reveals the lack of such resources.

Each of the three cycles of louse-borne relapsing fever in Sudan had distinct characteristics. Even from 1908 to 1925 Egyptians were the most frequent victims. The number of cases was few and the disease was easily controlled. From 1926 to 1932 the acute epidemic entered Darfur from the west, and the appearance of a mild form further east suggested that a concerted effort could keep the disease in check. The last phase, from 1936 to 1951, saw the disease enter from the east and become endemic throughout central Sudan. Adequate treatment prevented a great loss of human life. But if World War II had robbed Sudan of trained personnel or medicine for treating the disease, the loss of life could have been staggering. As it was, the conclusion of the war in 1945 enabled the Medical Service to acquire enough DDT powder to take the offensive against a worthy opponent, the louse.

Notes

1. There is disagreement on the issue of outside introduction; see R. Kirk, "The Epidemiology of Relapsing Fever in the Anglo-Egyptian Sudan," *Annals of Tropical Medicine and Parasitology*, XXXIII (1939), 130.

2. A brief discussion of the epidemic as well as a map illustrating its course is found in Erich Martini, "Globale Verbreitung der Läuse-Rückfallfieber," *Welt-Seuchen-Atlas/World-Atlas of Epidemic Disease*, Ernst Rodenwaldt, ed. (Hamburg, 1956), II, 53–54. Also see League of Nations, Health Section, "Relapsing Fever," *Fourth Epidemiological Report for 1926* (1927), pp. 22–24.

3. Charles Wilcocks and P. E. C. Manson-Bahr, eds., *Manson's Tropical Diseases* (Baltimore, 1972 edition), pp. 584–89; also see Anna C. Gelman, "The Ecology of the Relapsing Fevers," *Studies in Disease Ecology*, Jacques M. May, ed. (New York, 1961), pp. 113–36.

4. Kirk, "Epidemiology of Relapsing Fever," p. 129; H. C. Squires, *The Sudan Medical Service; An Experiment in Social Medicine* (London, 1958), pp. 41–43; G. K. Maurice, "The Entry of Relapsing Fever into the Sudan," *Sudan Notes and Records*, XV (1932), 98.

5. Maurice, "Entry of Relapsing Fever," p. 100.

6. Harold MacMichael, *The Anglo-Egyptian Sudan* (London, 1934), p. 221.

7. Maurice, "Entry of Relapsing Fever," pp. 97–118.

8. *Ibid.*, p. 101.

9. C. E. G. Beveridge, "The Louse-Borne Type of Relapsing Fever as Prevalent in the Anglo-Egyptian Sudan, 1926 and 1927," *The Medical Journal of Australia*, I (28 January 1928), 110.

10. Maurice, "Entry of Relapsing Fever," p. 101.

11. Nogue, "L'Épidémie de fièvre récurrente en Afrique occidentale française (1921–1924)," *Annales de médecine et de pharmacie coloniales*, XXIII (1925), 445ff., Rigollet, "Origine du typhus récurrent en Afrique occidentale française," *Bulletin de la société de pathologie exotique*, XVIII (1925), 679ff. P. S. Selwyn-Clarke, G. H. LeFanu, and A. Ingram, "Relapsing Fever in the Gold Coast," *Annals of Tropical Medicine and Parasitology*, XVII (1923), 389ff.

12. W. E. McCulloch, "Relapsing Fever in Northern Nigeria—a Study of 300 Cases," *Journal of Tropical Medicine and Hygiene,* XXVIII (1925), 334; also see N. A. Dyce Sharp, "Epidemic Disease in West Africa; The Menace of the Future," *Transactions of the Royal Society of Tropical Medicine and Hygiene,* XIX (1925–26), 256–64; relevant, but published later, is a communication about Sokoto district: P. J. Caffrey, "Relapsing Fever in Northern Nigeria, Some Observations," *Transactions of the Royal Society of Tropical Medicine and Hygiene,* XX (1926–27), 195–97.

13. Dr. LeGac, "L'Épidémie de fièvre récurrente au Ouadaï (Tchad), 1925–1928," *Annales de médecine et de pharmacie coloniales,* XXIX (1931), 150–51. One French official had thought of communicating with officials in Khartoum but he was not stationed in Africa nor was he responsible for such matters. He mused: "It would be interesting to know whether the Anglo-Egyptian Sudan has hitherto remained immune from the disease [relapsing fever] and whether special health agreements on this subject have been reached between that country and the Chad territory for the purpose of checking the spread of the epidemic." League of Nations, Health Organization, *Public Health Services in the French Colonies,* by S. Abbatucci, no. 3 (1926), 127; also see pp. 46–47.

14. Sudan, Ministry of Health, *Annual Report for 1926,* pp. 1–3.

15. *Ibid.,* p. 1.

16. Maurice, "Entry of Relapsing Fever," p. 110.

17. *Ibid.,* pp. 103–6.

18. *Annual Report for 1926,* p. 1.

19. *Ibid.,* p. 2.

20. *Annual Report for 1933,* p. 5.

21. Kirk, "The Epidemiology of Relapsing Fever," p. 130; see p. 126 also.

22. MacMichael, *The Anglo-Egyptian Sudan,* pp. 219, 221.

23. *Annual Report for 1933,* p. 4.

24. *Annual Report for 1926,* p. 2; the Director of the Sudan Medical Service subsequently used these same figures, O. P. H. Atkey, "L'Épidémie de fièvre récurrente au Soudan de 1926 a 1928," *Bulletin mensuel de l'office international d'hygiene publique,* XXI (1929), 1932; Atkey, "La fièvre récurrente au Soudan en 1930," *Bulletin mensuel de l'office international d'hygiene publique,* XXIII (1931), 2000–6.

25. D. Riding and T. W. MacDowell, "Preliminary Notes on Relapsing Fever in the Anglo-Egyptian Sudan," *Transactions of the Royal Society of Tropical Medicine and Hygiene,* XX (1926–27), 529.

26. Maurice, "The Entry of Relapsing Fever," p. 116. Zalingei District was one of five districts afflicted in Darfur, the other districts included Kebkebia, Nyala, Kuttum, and El Fasher. Thus other people besides the Fur suffered as well. In addition, the estimate of Zalingei's total population in 1926 seems low. In 1937 an estimate of 120,000 was given for Zalingei by A. C. Beaton in "The Fur," *Sudan Notes and Records,* XXIX (1948), 2. Beaton refers to the Fur in Zalingei District as the central Fur with two other sections living in neighboring districts.

27. *Ibid.,* p. 97.

28. *Annual Report for 1933,* p. 4. The last mortality estimates submitted by Anglo-Egyptian Sudan to the League of Nations were published in early 1927; thereafter only descriptions of progress in fighting the epidemic were submitted: League of Nations, Health Section, "The Relapsing-Fever Epidemic in Anglo-Egyptian Sudan," *Monthly Epidemiological Report* (15 February 1927), pp. 81–82.

29. Maurice, "The Entry of Relapsing Fever," p. 113.

30. *Ibid.*, p. 114.

31. *Ibid.*, p. 118. For remarks regarding the psychological, economic, and cultural consequences of Europe's encounter with plague see William H. McNeill, *Plagues and Peoples* (Garden City, N.Y., 1976), pp. 182–86.

32. The Republic of Sudan, H. Q. Council of Ministers, Department of Statistics, *First Population Census of Sudan, 1955/1956, Final Report,* vol. III (Khartoum, 1962), p. 117. Also see footnote 26.

33. League of Nations, "Relapsing Fever," p. 23.

34. *Annual Report for 1929,* p. 6.

35. *Annual Report for 1928,* p. 5; *Annual Report for 1929,* pp. 6–7.

36. Beveridge, "The Louse Borne Type of Relapsing Fever," p. 110. Beveridge's estimate was subsequently cited by David Scott in *Epidemic Disease in Ghana, 1901–1960* (London, 1965), p. 124, and also attributed to mortality in Sudan alone. But a careful reading of Beveridge's statement leaves one perplexed; the 200,000 figure could also be interpreted to be the estimated mortality from the beginning of the epidemic in 1921.

37. *Ibid.*, p. 112.

38. *Ibid.*, p. 110. The movement of people into and through Sudan, whether pilgrims or laborers, presents numerous health problems; see Ahmed Bayoumi, "Mecca Pilgrimage: The Socio-Medical Problems It Presents in the Sudan," *Sudan Medical Journal,* X, 2 (1972), 110; A. O. Abu Shamma, "International Aspects of Public Health," *The Health of the Sudan; A Study in Social Development,* H. Butler, ed. (Khartoum, 1963), pp. 101–3; A. Bukhari, "The Rural Health Service in the Sudan," *Sudan Medical Journal,* I, 4 (1956), 2.

39. Kirk, "The Epidemiology of Relapsing Fever," p. 128.

40. Such an interpretation is supported by Dr. LeGac on the Chadian side of the border as well; see "L'Épidémie de fièvre récurrente au Ouadaï," pp. 151–52.

41. Riding and MacDowell, "Preliminary Notes on Relapsing Fever," p. 525; Kirk, "The Epidemiology of Relapsing Fever," pp. 129–30.

42. Riding and MacDowell, "Preliminary Notes on Relapsing Fever," p. 526.

43. Maurice clearly supports this position as well; see "The Entry of Relapsing Fever," p. 114.

44. "Preliminary Notes on Relapsing Fever," p. 528.

45. "The Louse-Borne Type of Relapsing Fever," p. 111.

46. Kirk, "The Epidemiology of Relapsing Fever," p. 134.

47. LeGac, "L'Épidémie de fièvre récurrente," p. 148.

48. *Annual Report for 1926,* p. 2.

49. Maurice, "The Entry of Relapsing Fever," p. 113.

50. *Ibid.*, p. 114.

51. *Ibid.*

52. *Ibid.*, p. 115.

53. *Ibid.*

54. *Ibid.*, p. 116.

55. *Annual Report for 1926,* p. 3.

56. *Annual Report for 1927,* pp. 2–3.

57. Beveridge, "The Louse-Borne Type of Relapsing Fever," p. 112.

58. Riding and MacDowell, "Preliminary Notes on Relapsing Fever," p. 528.

59. *Annual Report for 1927,* p. 3.

60. *Ibid.*

61. *Annual Report for 1930,* pp. 9–10.

62. *Annual Report for 1933,* p. 5.

63. *Annual Report for 1937,* p. 6.

64. Kirk, "The Epidemiology of Relapsing Fever," p. 131.

65. *Ibid.*, pp. 134–35.

66. *Annual Report for 1937*, p. 5.

67. *Annual Report for 1938*, pp. 6–7.

68. *Ibid.*, p. 6.

69. *Ibid.*

70. Kirk, "The Epidemiology of Relapsing Fever," p. 137; *Annual Report for 1937*, p. 5.

71. Kirk, "The Epidemiology of Relapsing Fever," p. 138.

72. *Annual Report for 1938*, p. 7.

73. *Annual Report for 1939*, p. 7.

74. *Annual Report for 1940*, p. 5.

75. *Annual Report for 1944*, p. 2.

76. *Annual Report for 1945*, p. 3; *Annual Report for 1946*, p. 4. Although specifically referring to malaria and yellow fever, William H. McNeill's assessment of DDT's global impact is supported by this examination of relapsing fever and its vector, the louse: "The sudden lifting of the malarial burden brought about by liberal use of DDT in the years immediately after World War II was one of the most dramatic and abrupt health changes ever experienced by mankind." McNeill, *Plagues and Peoples*, p. 282.

77. Maurice, "Entry of Relapsing Fever," p. 118.

9

Bibliographical Essay

K. David Patterson

The range and diversity of the literature in this field is illustrated in the footnotes documenting the studies in this book. This brief essay, a condensed and updated version of a paper published in 1974,[1] is designed for persons interested in further reading or research. As in the original essay, coverage will be selective and restricted to material on sub-Saharan Africa.

Good, readable introductions to medical history and the nature of disease can be found in Charles Wilcocks, *Medical Advance, Public Health, and Social Evolution* (Oxford, 1965); F. M. Burnet and D. O. White, *Natural History of Infectious Disease* (Cambridge, 1965; 4th ed., 1972); and René Dubos, *Man Adapting* (New Haven, 1965). Charles Singer and E. A. Underwood's frequently cited *A Short History of Medicine* (2nd ed., Oxford, 1962) is a lengthy and encyclopedic compilation of scientific advances, mainly useful for reference. *A History of Tropical Medicine* by H. H. Scott (Baltimore, 1939, 2 vols.) is a basic source, and progress in understanding several organisms infesting Africans is described in William Derek Foster's *A History of Parasitology* (Edinburgh, 1965). George Rosen's *A History of Public Health* (New York, 1958) is a standard work which focuses on Western Europe and the United States, but it is essential reading for those interested in public health in Africa, especially in the cities. A classic study by August Hirsch, *Handbook of Geographical and Historical Pathology* (English edition, London, 1883–86, 3 vols.) is a gold mine of information on specific diseases and is an excellent guide to the older literature; a more modern work on the same subject is *History and Geography of the Most Im-*

portant Diseases (New York, 1965) by Edwin H. Ackerknecht.

Medical literature can be conveniently located in the invaluable *Index Medicus* published by the National Library of Medicine in Bethesda, Maryland. *The Index Catalogue of the Library of the Surgeon-General's Office* is useful for older materials. Research in all aspects of medical history can be followed in the National Library of Medicine's comprehensive annual *Bibliography of the History of Medicine* and in *Current Work in the History of Medicine: An International Bibliography,* published by the Wellcome Institute of the History of Medicine. Short but useful introductions to the medical literature on Africa are Charles Wilcocks, "Some Sources of Information on Tropical Medicine" (*International Review of Tropical Medicine,* I, 1961, 269–83) and especially Charles Tettey, "Medicine in Africa: A Bibliographical Essay" (*Current Bibliography of African Affairs,* January 1970, 5–18). Tettey's *Medicine in British West Africa, 1880–1956, An Annotated Bibliography* (Accra, 1975) is extremely helpful. Important summaries of health conditions and medical services in the various colonial empires are found in Lord Hailey, *An African Survey* (London, 1938; revised ed., 1957) and E. B. Worthington, *Science in Africa: A Review of Scientific Research Relating to Tropical and South Africa* (London, 1938).

Historians of medicine have subjected their discipline to extensive self-examination in recent years. For example, Edwin Clarke has edited a collection of essays entitled *Modern Methods in the History of Medicine* (London, 1971), which he describes as a "manifesto" to those seeking new approaches and a higher standard of research and writing. An essay by Mary Boas Hall, "History of Science and History of Medicine," argues that both fields have suffered from a lack of professionalism and a tendency to interpret theories and controversies of the past from the perspective of present knowledge. Charles Rosenberg's contribution to the collection, "The Medical Profession, Medical Practice, and the History of Medicine," urges a shift in emphasis from a history of technical and theoretical advance to medicine as actually practiced; from medical "high culture" to the impact of medicine on daily life. Thomas McKeown, in "A Sociological Approach to the History of Medicine" (*Medical History,* XIV, 1970, 342–51), asserts that medical history "takes its terms of reference from problems confronting medicine in the present day." He suggests research on health care systems, public health, and the development of hospitals, topics certainly significant for Africanists. Gerald N. Grob's "The Social History of Medicine and Disease in America: Problems and Possibilities" (*Journal of Social History,* X, 1977, 391–409) raises issues which should concern historians of Africa as well as those of the United States. These and similar writings should dispel any lingering fears that an interest in medical history implies a proclivity toward irrelevant antiquarianism.

Studies on other parts of the world suggest issues which should be examined in Africa. Hans Zinsser's inimitable *Rats, Lice, and History* (New York, 1935, and many subsequent editions) is informative and amusing. William H. McNeill's *Plagues and Peoples* (New York, 1976) is a bold, provocative, and well-written introduction to the interrelationships between disease and world history; it deserves a wide and careful readership. Unfortunately, because of the limited research done so far, McNeill can say relatively little about Africa. Thomas McKeown's important research on European demographic history, presented in several articles and in *The Modern Rise of Population* (New York, 1976), shows that better nutrition and sanitation were much more important than the activities of doctors in mortality reduction in Western societies. This is not necessarily the case in modern Africa, where medical measures have probably played a larger role. Epidemics have periodically swept African societies and, as Asa Briggs suggests in his stimulating article "Cholera and Society in the Nineteenth Century" (*Past and Present,* XIX, 1961, 76–96), a severe epidemic tests existing political, social, economic, and religious systems. Case studies of general interest include Donald B. Cooper, *Epidemic Disease in Mexico City, 1761–1813: An Administrative, Social, and Medical Study* (Austin, 1965); John Duffy, *Sword of Pestilence: The New Orleans Yellow Fever Epidemic of 1853* (Baton Rouge, 1966): Roderick

E. McGrew, *Russia and the Cholera, 1823–1832* (Madison, 1965); and Charles E. Rosenberg, *The Cholera Years: The United States in 1832, 1849, and 1866* (Chicago, 1962).

Any consideration of disease and medicine in Africa must of course consider local theories and cures, even though present health conditions on the continent suggest that indigenous medical systems were relatively ineffectual. No attempt will be made to survey the extensive and growing literature of medical anthropology, but three important books, classics in the field, must be cited. These are Margaret J. Field's pioneering work on the Gold Coast, *Religion and Medicine of the Ga People* (New York, 1937), *Native African Medicine: With Special Reference to its Practice in the Mano Tribe of Liberia* (Cambridge, Mass., 1941; reprinted London, 1970) by George Way Harley, and Michael Gelfand's *Witch Doctor: Traditional Medicine Man of Rhodesia* (London, 1964), a study of Shona healers. Harley and Gelfand are physicians sympathetic to some African psychological and pharmaceutical practices. The close relationship between religion and healing is further documented in Frederick Quinn "How Traditional Dahomian Society Interpreted Smallpox" (*Abbia,* XX, 1968, 151–66), while the vast extent of some African pharmacopoeias is illustrated by Abbé André Raponda Walker and Roger Sillans in their massive *Les Plantes utiles du Gabon* (Paris, 1961). Historical studies of indigenous medicine are possible for a few societies with long literary traditions. For example, Stefan Strelcyn has examined classic Ge'ez medical texts in "Les Ecrits médicaux éthiopiens" (*Journal of Ethiopian Studies,* III, 1965, 82–103), and Ismail Hussein Abdalla is studying the history of Arabic medical influence on Hausa practitioners (University of Wisconsin doctoral dissertation, in progress).

The findings of medical anthropologists are of course essential to any consideration of African responses to western medicine. Although largely theoretical, *Adaptation in Cultural Evolution: An Approach to Medical Anthropology* (New York, 1970) by Alexander Alland, Jr., contains interesting material on the medical system of the Abron of the Ivory Coast and its response to government and missionary health efforts. Una Maclean's short book, *Magical Medicine: A Nigerian Case Study* (London, 1971) is even more illuminating. Her fascinating study of popular medicine in Ibadan explores the adaptations of "traditional" Yoruba medicine to modern urban conditions and competition between two very different types of health care. Possible consequences of overenthusiastic adoption of modern techniques are gruesomely illustrated in David R. Fry's "Some Complications of Illicit Injections (West Cameroon)" (*West African Medical Journal,* XIV, 1965, 167–69).

The medical history of precolonial Africa is still an almost entirely unexplored field, but a few signposts do exist. Philip Curtin's seminal study of the impact of infectious diseases on the South Atlantic economic system, "Epidemiology and the Slave Trade" (*Political Science Quarterly,* LXXXIII, 1968, 190–216), shows that movements of peoples among the discrete disease environments of Europe, Africa, and the Americas had major consequences. His suggestion that African populations suffered from epidemics as isolation was broken down seems valid for early trade contacts as well as for the initial phases of colonial expansion. Alfred W. Crosby treats the interchange of pathogens and crops in an authoritative and readable style in *The Columbian Exchange: The Biological and Cultural Consequences of 1492* (Westport, Conn., 1972). The focus is on the Western Hemisphere, but there is some material on Africa. Any work on the history of diseases in coastal West Africa will depend heavily on R. Hoeppli's well-researched monograph, *Parasitic Diseases in Africa and the Western Hemisphere: Early Documentation and Transmission by the Slave Trade* (*Acta Tropica,* suppl. 10, Basel, 1969).

Several short studies of particular problems and regions should also be noted. R. Hoeppli has collaborated with C. Lucasse to show the antiquity of trypanosomiasis in "Old Ideas Regarding Cause and Treatment of Sleeping Sickness Held in West Africa" (*Journal of Tropical Medicine and Hygiene,* LXVII, 1964, 60–68). An outline of Portuguese health measures in Angola prior to 1844 is available in "Subsidos para a historia da medicina em Angola (até à organização do serviço de saude)" (*Boletim do*

Instituto de Angola, XXX/XXXII, 1968, 5–26) by Waldemar Jorges Gomes Teixeira. Among the voluminous writings of Richard Pankhurst are several interesting contributions to the medical history of Ethiopia, including "The History of Famine and Pestilence in Ethiopia Prior to the Founding of Gondar" (*Journal of Ethiopian Studies,* X, 1972, 37–64), "Some Factors Influencing the Health of Traditional Ethiopia" (*Journal of Ethiopian Studies,* IV, 1966, 31–70), "Old Time Ethiopian Cures for Syphilis, Seventeenth to Nineteenth Centuries" (*Journal of the History of Medicine and Allied Sciences,* XXX, 1975, 199–216), and "The History and Traditional Treatment of Smallpox in Ethiopia" (*Medical History,* IX, 1965, 343–55). The last article describes variolization and the encouragement of vaccination by Menelik.

The history of famines in Africa is, unfortunately, a timely topic. Pankhurst has made a perceptive analysis of the course and consequences of one disaster in "The Great Ethiopian Famine of 1888–1892: A New Assessment" (*Journal of the History of Medicine,* XXI, 1966, 95–124 and 271–94). "The Heritage of Famine in Central Tanzania" is briefly sketched from the mid-nineteenth century until independence by Clarke Brooke (*Tanzania Notes and Records,* LXVII, 1967, 15–22). Sèkéné-Mody Cissoko has used indigenous sources to describe "Famines et épidémies à Tombouctou et dans la Boucle du Niger du XVIe au XVIIIe siècle" (*Bulletin de l'Institut Fondamental d'Afrique Noire,* sér. B, XXX, 1968, 806–21). However, his gloomy account of the calamities of the post-1951 period seems exaggerated; Cissko appears to share the pro-Songhai bias of the chroniclers who provide his data. A twentieth-century famine is described in Finn Fuglestad, "La grande famine de 1931 dans l'ouest nigérien: réflexions autour d'une catastrophe naturelle" (*Revue française d'histoire d'outre-mer,* 61, 1974, 18–33).

Writings on recent African medical history are, as might be expected, much more numerous than for the precolonial era. But, despite much better source materials, the quality of work on the colonial period is not necessarily higher. A common format for twentieth-century studies is *A History of Medicine in Territory X,* usually assembled by a physician with long years of experience in Territory X. These books tend to be stodgy narratives of administrative developments, frequently interrupted by personal anecdotes and laudatory capsule biographies of any health worker who ever set foot in X. Such works nonetheless contain a wealth of information and, as amateurs in history are more useful and presumably less dangerous than amateurs in medicine, their production is a real contribution. A work by the late Percy Ward Laidler and Michael Gelfand, *South Africa: Its Medical History, 1652–1898* (Cape Town, 1971) is almost a caricature of this genre. It rambles over a vast amount of undigested material with little evidence of selectivity; anything the authors found seems to have been stuck in somewhere. However, despite its distinctly antiquarian flavor, the volume is loaded with data on medical and social history and suggests many topics for professional treatment. Edmund H. Burrows deals with the same subject much more coherently. *A History of Medicine in South Africa up to the End of the Nineteenth Century* (Cape Town, 1958) is, like the previously cited volume, almost totally Eurocentric, but contains some interesting material on Boer folk medicine. Ann Beck has covered some fairly dreary material in *A History of British Medical Administration of East Africa, 1900–1950* (Cambridge, Mass., 1970). Professor Beck has also published "The Role of Medicine in German East Africa" (*Bulletin of the History of Medicine,* XLV, 1971, 170–78), "The East African Community and Regional Research in Science and Medicine" (*African Affairs,* LXXII, 1973, 300–308), and *Medicine and Society in Tanganyika, 1890–1930: A Historical Inquiry* (Philadelphia, 1977). One of the better works of its kind is David F. Clyde's detailed *History of the Medical Services of Tanganyika* (Dar-es-Salaam, 1962); it is, however, largely administrative history with extensive coverage of World War I. *The Early History of Scientific Medicine in Uganda* (Nairobi, 1970), a short book by William Derek Foster, is a modest but well-done study of the 1870–1910 period. The title of H. C. Squire's *The Sudan Medical Service: An Experiment in Social Medicine* (London, 1958) promises more than is delivered, but there is a useful discussion of Sudanese medical education. A. Bayoumi's account of "Medical Research in the

Sudan since 1903" (*Medical History*, XIX, 1975, 271–85) is also interesting. "The Beginnings of Modern Medicine in Ethiopia" from the travels of James Bruce until the Italian invasion are described in colorful detail by Richard Pankhurst (*Ethiopia Observer*, IX, 1965, 114–60). Pankhurst's writings on Ethiopia are matched in volume by Michael Gelfand's studies of the territories which once comprised British Central Africa. Gelfand's first book, a popular publication dedicated to Cecil Rhodes, shows his strong prosettler bias. *Tropical Victory: An Account of the Influence of Medicine on the History of Southern Rhodesia, 1890–1923* (Cape Town, 1953) does, however, illustrate how important medical technology was for the success of white colonization. Gelfand's later historical works, *Northern Rhodesia in the Days of the Charter: A Medical and Social Study, 1878–1924* (Oxford, 1961) and *Lakeside Pioneers: Socio-Medical Study of Nyasaland (1875–1920)* (Oxford, 1965), are much more substantial but have relatively little to say about Africans. This is partially remedied in *A Service to the Sick: A History of the Health Services for Africans in Southern Rhodesia (1890–1953)* (Guelo, Rhodesia, 1976). Colin Baker's "The Government Medical Service in Malawi, An Administrative History 1891–1974" (*Medical History*, XX, 1976, 296–311) should also be noted.

Less writing of this kind has been done on West Africa, except for a massive, amateurish, but welcome volume by Ralph Schram, *A History of the Nigerian Health Services* (Ibadan, 1971). Thomas S. Gale has described the development of the West African Medical Service in his doctoral dissertation *Official Medical Policy in British West Africa, 1870–1930* (University of London, School of Oriental and African Studies, 1973) and has attacked, justly, the health policies of a leading colonial figure in "Lord F. D. Lugard: An Assessment of His Contributions to Medical Policy in Nigeria" (*International Journal of African Historical Studies*, IX, 1976, 631–40). In a rather different vein is Dr. Adelola Adeloye's article, "Some Early Nigerian Doctors and Their Contributions to Modern Medicine in West Africa" (*Medical History*, XVIII, 1974, 275–93). There is some historical material on the French colonies in M. Sankale's *Médicine et ac-*

tion sanitaire en Afrique noire (Paris, 1969). An older work by C. Mathis, *L'Oeuvre des pastoriens en Afrique noire: Afrique Occidentale Française* (Paris, 1946), is also useful. Finally, Charles Tettey has described a vital but chronically under-financed and understaffed aspect of colonial health care in "A Brief History of the Medical Research Institute and Laboratory Service of the Gold Coast (Ghana), 1908–1957." (*West African Medical Journal*, IX, 1960, 73–85). Liberia has so far been ignored.

The medical and veterinary importance of trypanosome infections forced colonial governments to undertake major research and control activities. The technical literature on this subject is vast and sleeping sickness has been the focus of several historical investigations. Two recent books by scientists with long experience in efforts to combat the disease provide superb introductions to this complex but fascinating field. John Ford's *The Role of the Trypanosomiases in African Ecology: A Study of the Tsetse Fly Problem* (Oxford, 1971) is a large and somewhat difficult work, with a strong emphasis on ecological and historical factors. He argues persuasively that human sleeping sickness was long endemic in East Africa and that it appeared in epidemic form as a result of socioenvironmental changes associated with the early colonial period. Trypanosomes, tsetses, and control measures are described in Rhodesia and Nigeria, as well as East Africa. John J. McKelvey, Jr., has written an equally valuable but quite different book, *Man Against Tsetse: Struggle for Africa* (Ithaca, 1973). As the title suggests, it is a more general work and presents less difficulty to historians and other nonspecialists. Written in a clear and lively style, it presents the basic biological data and describes major campaigns against the disease, including Portuguese efforts on Principe Island, Eugène Jamot's paramilitary operations in Cameroun and French West Africa, and the Anchau scheme in Northern Nigeria. Because control measures often involved extensive surveys and major social engineering by colonial governments, records of such campaigns may contain valuable data for social and economic historians. Both Ford and McKelvey provide extensive bibliographies.

Several other studies on sleeping sickness should be noted. K. R. S. Morris argues that the disease was spread from western to eastern Africa as a result of greater human mobility in the late nineteenth century in "The Movement of Sleeping Sickness Across Central Africa" (*Journal of Tropical Medicine and Hygiene*, LXVI, 1963, 59–76). The disastrous Ugandan epidemic is described by Ford and McKelvey and in Foster's book on Ugandan medicine, as well as in works by B. W. Langlands, *The Sleeping Sickness Epidemic of Uganda 1900–1920: A Study in Historical Geography* (Kampala, 1967), and Harvey G. Soff, "Sleeping Sickness in the Lake Victoria Region of British East Africa, 1900–1915" (*African Historical Studies*, II, 1969, 255–68). Soff extends his coverage in his Syracuse University doctoral dissertation, *A History of Sleeping Sickness in Uganda: Administrative Response 1900–1970* (1971). Charles M. Good discusses the growth of trade as a factor in the spread of sleeping sickness and relapsing fever in "Salt, Trade, and Disease: Aspects of Development in Africa's Northern Great Lakes Region" (*International Journal of African Historical Studies*, V, 1972, 543–86). A. J. Duggan's "A Survey of Sleeping Sickness in Northern Nigeria from the Earliest Times to the Present Day" (*Transactions of the Royal Society of Tropical Medicine and Hygiene*, LVI, 1962, 439–86) places greater emphasis than Ford on the *Pax Brittanica* as a factor in the spread of the disease. Duggan has also written a suggestive local study which deftly incorporates historical, ethnographic, and ecological factors, "The Occurrence of Human Trypanosomiasis Among the Rukuba Tribe of Northern Nigeria" (*Journal of Tropical Medicine and Hygiene*, LXV, 1962, 151–63). Leroy Vail's fine article, "Ecology and History: The Example of Eastern Zambia" (*Journal of Southern African Studies*, III, 1977, 129–55) describes the effects of social change and colonial policies on human and bovine trypanosomiasis and other diseases. As the title suggests, Vail also deals with such topics as wild animals, soil erosion, and declining agricultural productivity; his holistic approach deserves emulation.

Other diseases and epidemics have attracted much less attention, but some useful work has been done. An epidemiologist,

David Scott, surveys outbreaks of plague, yellow fever, smallpox, cerebrospinal meningitis, relapsing fever, trypanosomiasis, and influenza, and describes medical countermeasures in an important country in *Epidemic Disease in Ghana 1901–1960* (London, 1965). This is a very useful book, but perhaps because Scott did not use district and provincial level archives, it does not adequately assess the impact of these epidemics on Ghanaian peoples.

A periodic scourge of the Sudanic belt is discussed in a two-part article by B. Waddy, "African Epidemic Cerebro-Spinal Meningitis" (*Journal of Tropical Medicine and Hygiene*, LX, 1957, 179–89 and 218–23), but a historical study of its effects is needed. Similarly, little work has been done on smallpox, a disease which should have been relatively easy for colonial governments to control. Douglas L. Wheeler has contributed "A Note on Smallpox in Angola 1670–1875" (*Studia*, XIII/XIV, 1964, 351–62). Eugenia W. Herbert's study, "Smallpox Innoculation in Africa," *Journal of African History*, XVI, 1975, 539–59) shows variolization was a widespread practice in precolonial times. One wonders if this made colonial vaccination campaigns any more or less acceptable. "The Eradication of Smallpox" by Donald A. Henderson (*Scientific American*, CCXXXV, October 1976, 25–33) describes the hopefully complete success of modern control methods. Good sources on malaria, Africa's most critical health problem, are Michael J. Colbourne, *Malaria in Africa* (London, 1966), and R. Mansell Prothero, *Migrants and Malaria* (London, 1965). Despite the importance of helminthic infections, little historical work has been done on them, with the happy exception of F. R. Sandbach's "The History of Schistosomiasis Research and Policy for Its Control" (*Medical History*, XX, 1976, 259–75).

Studies of African epidemics are still scarce, and they are not all new. James Christie's pioneering *Cholera Epidemics in East Africa* (London, 1876; reprinted London, 1970) is a significant historical source for the whole region. His detailed account of health conditions in Zanzibar and the ravages of cholera there suggests that the medical history of this cosmopolitan commercial entrepot is accessible and important. C. Van Onselen describes a major epizootic and analyzes its political, economic, and social impact in an excellent study, "Reactions to Rinderpest in Southern Africa, 1896–1897" (*Journal of African History*, XIII, 1972, 473–88). A pair of articles show how yellow fever could influence colonial policy. Claude Pulvenis depicts the helplessness of the French in the face of an epidemic in Senegal and how the push to the Niger was temporarily disrupted by heavy European mortality in "Une Epidémie de fièvre jaune à Saint-Louis du Sénégal (1881)" (*Bulletin de l'Institut Fondamental d'Afrique Noire*, sér. B, XXX, 1968, 1353–73). Christophe Wondji's "La Fièvre jaune à Grand Bassam (1899–1903)" (*Revue française d'histoire d'outre-mer*, LIX, 1972, 205–39) describes the health problems of that Ivorien town, which were partly responsible for shifting the colonial capital to Bingerville. The influenza pandemic of 1918–19, one of the most devastating episodes in the demographic history of Africa, has begun to attract scholarly interest. I. R. Phimster's "The 'Spanish' Influenza Pandemic of 1918 and its Impact on the Southern Rhodesian Mining Industry" (*Central African Medical Journal*, XIX, 1973, 143–48), Richard Pankhurst's "The Hedar Basita of 1918" (*Journal of Ethiopian Studies*, XIII, 1975, 103–31), and K. David Patterson's "The Influenza Epidemic of 1918–19 in the Gold Coast" (to appear in *Transactions of the Historical Society of Ghana*, XVI, 1977) suggest the magnitude of the disaster.

Some political implications of colonial medical policies are described in Leo Spitzer's essay, "The Mosquito and Segregation in Sierra Leone" (*Canadian Journal of African Studies*, II, 1968, 49–61) and in an important contribution by Raymond E. Dumett, "The Campaign Against Malaria and the Expansion of Scientific Medical and Sanitary Services in British West Africa, 1898–1910" (*African Historical Studies*, I, 1968, 153–97). N. R. E. Fendall's "A History of the Yaba School of Medicine, Nigeria" (*West African Medical Journal*, XVI, 1967, 118–24) is a useful treatment of neglected subject. B. B. Waddy, a veteran British health officer, criticizes the absence of intercolonial medical cooperation in his essay "Frontiers and Disease in West Africa" (*Journal of Tropical Medicine and Hygiene*, LXI, 1958, 100–107). The article raises questions about general relations between French and British colonial administrations and the possible special problems or opportunities of Africans living in border areas.

Historians will find much continuity with the past in descriptions of current health problems and debates over how to solve them. Good general surveys are found in L. Dudley Stamp, *Africa, A Study in Tropical Development* (2nd ed., New York, 1966) and in volume II of George H. T. Kimble's *Tropical Africa* (New York, 1960). Waddy summarizes the postindependence situation in the West African interior in "The Present State of Public Health in the African Soudan" (*Transactions of the Royal Society of Tropical Medicine and Hygiene*, LVI, 1962, 95–115). R. Cook's "The General Nutritional Problems of Africa" (*African Affairs*, LXV, 1966, 329–40) is a good overview. Debates over the role of paramedical staff were common in the colonial period and continue today. The case for greater utilization of such persons is made by N. R. E. Fendall in "The Medical Assistant in Africa" (*Journal of Tropical Medicine and Hygiene*, LXXI, 1968, 83–95). Slightly different approaches to the vital needs of rural health care are found in M. Sankale, *Médicine et action sanitaire en Afrique noire* (Paris, 1969) and Maurice King, ed., *Medical Care in Developing Countries: A Primer on the Medicine of Poverty* (London, 1966). M. J. Sharpston examines a common but critical problem in "Uneven Geographical Distribution of Medical Care: A Ghanaian Case Study" (*Journal of Development Studies*, VIII, 1972, 205–22). It would be interesting to see if independent governments have done any better than colonial regimes in making medical care available throughout their territories. Unforeseen health problems caused by economic development projects are described in a superb review by Charles C. Hughes and John M. Hunter, "Disease and 'Development' in Africa" (*Social Science and Medicine*, III, 1970, 443–93), which should be required reading for all concerned with modernization schemes, past, present, or future.

1. "Disease and Medicine in African History: A Bibliographical Essay," *History in Africa*, 1 (1974), 141–48. Portions reprinted by permission.

Index